EAT to Your Good Health

EAT To Your Good Health: Exchange Lists & Meal Planning for Eating Disorders

Amy Galena, MSH, RD, LD/N

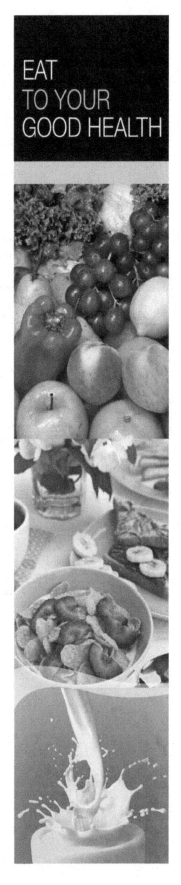

iUniverse, Inc.
Bloomington

Eat to Your Good Health
Exchange Lists and Meal Planning for Eating Disorders

iUniverse books may be ordered through booksellers or by contacting:

iUniverse
1663 Liberty Drive
Bloomington, IN 47403
www.iuniverse.com
1-800-Authors (1-800-288-4677)

ISBN: 978-1-4620-5531-9 (sc)
ISBN: 978-1-4620-5532-6 (e)

Printed in the United States of America

iUniverse rev. date: 2/26/2013

Foreword

The pressure for people to be and look perfect is at an all time high. It's mounting at an unparalleled pace. The media, society, and pop culture are playing a significant role in how people perceive themselves as beautiful or ugly. The perception is largely based on the features of a handful of super-models. The assumption is that everyone should look like that man or woman strutting down the run way. Technology has progressed so quickly in the last 30 years, and so has the way people communicate at a lightning fast pace. Since information travels so fast today, we are constantly being affected by worldwide perceptions of beauty and perfection.

Amy's booklet helps people understand that food is medicine not a poison to be avoided just to be thin. Within these pages is hope, a hope that they don't have to be afraid of food anymore. Hope that you already have the power to become the man or woman you choose to be. It also allows them come to the understanding that they are in charge of their health. The definition of nutrient rich foods is clearly explained and lots of easy to read charts are given to make living healthy accessible. This booklet hands each person their power back to live a healthy life style.

Be courageous! Courage is plugging into your truth when you feel discouraged or afraid. I invite you to start your own journey now. Create the fun, passionate, and vibrant life you've always wanted. It is possible to change your life one thought, action, and habit at a time.

~ Sarah E. Suero
Owner of Grounded and Company
Yoga Instructor, Ontological Coach, and Writer

EAT to Your Good Health Edited by Sarah E. Suero

Preface

"Don't wait for something big to occur. Start with where you are, with what you have, and that will always lead you into something greater." Mary Morrissey

When you read *EAT to Your Good Health*, I ask for you to think of food as medicine and to be honest with yourself. Acknowledge the state of your physical, dietary, and mental health. Here is your chance to learn to live vibrantly. Start making the right changes now and travel along the road towards true happiness.

I was in high school when I realized that my health was my choice. Everything that I ate and did was my choice. I educated myself on what it meant to live a healthy lifestyle and I changed accordingly. I ate nutrient rich foods, became more active, and created balance in my life. I began to feel much better. The shifts I made improved my energy, concentration, and happiness. I gained a positive outlook on life. I felt vibrant and in good mental and physical health. What I discovered was amazing; I could eat to my good health. I am so excited about my discoveries that I just have to share it with the world. I've never stopped my pursuit of a healthy lifestyle.

Now my mission is that each person thrives. Eat to your good health, so that you live out your dreams. I now teach people to live vibrantly, not just survive. My passion for food and health drove me to get my Master's in Health Science. As a lead dietitian in behavioral health and years of child/adolescent weight management work experience, I've realized everyone can be healthy. Due to that realization many years ago, I am now living my dream. I'm the proud owner of Bee Nutritious, an established business specializing in eating disorders. I wrote *EAT to Your Good Health* as a tool to help you along your journey. *EAT to Your Good Health* can help you develop a positive relationship with yourself and your food. Stop fighting nature and accept your body. The power is now in your hands.

Live Vibrantly,

~ Amy Galena

Acknowledgements

I'd like to take a few moments to thank several important people in my life. I appreciate each one for the value they bring to my life, the health community, and the world.

Thank you to Dr. Vaghefi for providing me with my first writing opportunity, which paved the way for many future opportunities and publications. You have been an incredible mentor in the fields of research and writing. Through your help and guidance I have come to improve my skills and career, and now I have written my first book. Thanks Dr. Vaghefi.

Thank you to Dr. Christie for being a steady rock of advice and guidance whenever I'm in need. You role model all that can be expected of a dietetic professional, and I will always admire you. Thanks Dr. Christie.

Thank you to Jon McGowan for your love and support that I needed to complete this booklet. You've always pushed me to be the best that I can be in life. I have learned so much from you over the years. I love you.

Acknowledgements

Contents

INTRODUCTION

EAT
TO YOUR
GOOD HEALTH

INTRODUCTION

HOW DO I USE *EAT TO YOUR GOOD HEALTH*?

EAT to Your Good Health provides exchange lists for meal planning, and essential nutrition education to promote healthy eating habits. Your registered dietitian will work with you to develop a meal plan that best suits your needs. A healthy meal plan includes carbohydrate, fruit, vegetables, dairy, fat, protein, and dessert. You may not be required to include all these foods each day in the very beginning, but eventually you and your dietitian will work together to incorporate all foods into your meal plan. *EAT to Your Good Health* is intended to coincide with regular nutrition counseling, which is vital to keep you on the path towards recovery.

WHAT DOES IT MEAN TO BE HEALTHY?

Good health is more than just being free from disease or injury. A healthy lifestyle helps you feel good, have vibrant energy, and maintain a positive outlook on life. A healthy lifestyle includes having physical, mental, and social well-being. Eating well, exercising properly, maintaining a healthy weight, staying positive, and having balance in your life all promote good health. The quality of life that you're creating ultimately depends on your choices. Your mental health is just as important as your physical health, and work together hand-and-hand. Letting go of your eating disorder, is one of the many ways to move towards good health.

WHAT IS HEALTHY EATING?

Healthy eating is consuming the right amounts of a variety of foods from all food groups to obtain the nutrients that your body needs to function at its best. Healthy eating promotes a vibrant and fully functioning mind and body. Healthy eating also helps fight off chronic diseases such as heart disease, diabetes, cancer, and osteoporosis.

WHAT IS AN EATING DISORDER?

An eating disorder is a condition in which self-destructive eating behaviors compromise your physical and mental health. Self-destructive eating behaviors include restricting food, binging, purging, laxative abuse, and compulsive exercise among others. An eating disorder also includes your beliefs about food and how they impact your body.

WHAT ARE SOME DANGERS OF EATING DISORDERS?

- Malnutrition
- Ruptured stomach (gastric rupture due to binge eating results in an 80% fatality rate)
- Serious heart, kidney and liver damage
- Internal bleeding
- Esophageal tears (throat tears) and rupture from vomiting
- Depression, anxiety, obsessive-compulsive disorder and substance abuse
- Tooth erosion/gum disease
- Low self-esteem
- Isolation and impaired social relationships
- Mood swings

- Constipation
- Muscle loss
- Osteoporosis
- Stunted growth
- Reduced metabolic rate
- Electrolyte imbalance
- Critically low blood pressure
- Irregular and/or low heart rate
- Cardiac arrest
- Death

EXERCISE AND EATING DISORDERS

Exercise is a great way to practice healthy living when it is done correctly. Exercise is important because it helps you feel good and maintain your natural body weight. Exercise is any form of physical body movement. There are many ways to become physically fit without harming you body. Intense exercise without a healthy approach to your nutrition is a form of purging. If you are currently under treatment for an eating disorder your exercise may be restricted, limited, and/or monitored due to your current medical and mental state. Following your meal plan, getting medically stable if needed, and decreasing your eating disorder behaviors are the best ways to gain back exercise if it has been restricted.

READINESS AND CONFIDENCE

You are in fact the author of your life, and you choose how you would like to live. There are many people that say they want to be healthy, but not all people are willing to do the work to being healthy. Frankly, healthiness is a lifestyle, not a diet plan to follow for a few months. I invite you to take a look at the scales below. Be honest with yourself, it's truly the only way to move through this eating disorder and into creating a vibrant life.

Directions: Complete the Readiness and Confidence Scales below. Discuss with your dietitian why you chose the numbers you did, and why you did not choose a different number. For example, if you circled a 5 or 6 than why did you choose that number instead of an 8, 9, or 10. Or if you choose a 10, than why did you choose a 10 instead of 9? There are blank journal pages at the back of *EAT to Your Good Health*. If you need to write more after finishing the scales, then do it.

Readiness

How ready are you to begin treatment, make positive changes, follow a meal plan, and start to let go of your eating disorder? 1 is feeling the "No, I'm not ready" and 10 "Yes, let's start today!"
Circle the number below that honestly reflects where you are.

Readiness scale

1	2	3	4	5	6	7	8	9	10

Confidence

How confident are you that you can do it? 1 is feeling, "No, I can't do it" and 10 is feeling, "Yes, I can! There isn't anyone that could stop me!"

Circle the number below that honestly reflects where you are.

Confidence scale

1	2	3	4	5	6	7	8	9	10

HOW DOES MEAL PLANNING WORK?

Your meal plan: The plan will incorporate exchanges from different food groups to meet your recommended calorie goal, which is set by your dietitian. Your calorie goal is calculated according to six areas: your height, weight, activity level, sex, age, and current food intake. Your meal plan will include at least three meals and one snack per day. Your dietitian will work with you to not obsess about calories. This may take some work. For that reason, calories have been left off the exchanges lists and will not be discussed in *EAT to Your Good Health*.

Do not skip meals. Your meal plan is part of your prescription. Think of your meal plan like a prescription medication for an illness or disease. When you are sick or not feeling well and go to the doctor, the doctor prescribes medicine that you need to take to become well. You must follow your meal plan and not skip any meals in order to feel better and be healthy. Skipping meals, especially breakfast can set you up for failure!

10 reasons why skipping meals is not a healthy diet practice:
- May cause you to become too hungry and overeat at your next meal
- May cause you to have cravings for less healthier foods
- Slows your metabolism
- Reduces your energy
- Results in missed nutrients that your body needs
- Starves your brain, body, and muscles
- Disrupts your body's hunger satiety signals
- Can make it hard to concentrate and focus
- May cause irritability
- Slows process of recovery

IMPORTANT NOTE: As summarized by our government's Food and Nutrition Service, children who are breakfast eaters versus children who are non-breakfast eaters have a healthier body mass index, a healthier nutritional intake, a better academic success rate, a more positive mood, less behavior problems, superior focus and concentration, fewer illnesses, and better school attendance.[1]

---

[1] FNS. (Updated 21 February 2012) *Expanding school breakfast talking points.* [online] Available at: http://www.fns.usda.gov/cnd/breakfast/expansion/breakfast_talkingpoints.pdf. [Accessed 22 June 2012].

EXCHANGES

Exchanges help make meal planning simpler by categorizing foods into caloric equivalents. Exchanges allow equal food substitutions within the same food category. For example, 1 slice of bread can be substituted for ⅓ cup of rice or ½ cup of grits because all equal 1 starch exchange. Your dietitian will help you learn the exchange system.

Sometimes portion sizes can be deceiving because they may look bigger or smaller than they really are. Trust your dietitian and know that she/he has your best interests in mind. If you feel uncomfortable about your meal plan, then make sure you clearly communicate that to your dietitian. It is better to let your dietitian know what you are capable of doing instead of accepting the meal plan while knowing that you honestly cannot follow it. Keep in mind that your dietitian may push you to eat more, eat less, try new foods, or take away foods. Follow these changes while being honest with yourself and your dietitian.

Many foods such as soup, egg substitute, fat-free cheese, sugar-free Jell-O, and fat-free Cool Whip are not listed on *EAT to Your Good Health*'s exchange lists for a reason. *EAT to Your Good Health* does not advise people recovering from eating disorders include "diet" foods on their meal plan. Any food that implies a weight loss message is considered a "diet" food. Weight control bars/shakes, diet Jell-O, diet cereal, sugar-free or diet desserts, and most Special K products are considered "diet" foods. You need to learn how to incorporate all foods except "diet" foods into your diet. A healthy diet includes fried foods, desserts, and pizza when balanced with fruit, vegetables, and whole grains.

WATER

Water is essential for life. Water helps circulate nutrients, remove waste, and regulate your body temperature. Milk, juice, tea, and many other fluids may be counted towards your fluid intake. Be aware if you restricting fluid and/or losing fluid through purging or excretion you are at greater risk for dehydration. Make sure to drink enough fluids to keep your body running smoothly.

FOOD PREPARATION

In the beginning of treatment, it is a good idea to measure your foods. If your treatment or support team believes that you will have difficulty measuring the correct amount of food, then you will need someone else to measure and prepare your food for you. Eventually, you will learn to eyeball and "guesstimate" food measurements and become less rigid in your food preparation.

Some measurement abbreviations include:
Tbsp = tablespoon
tsp = teaspoon
oz = ounce
g = gram(s)
pcs = pieces

IMPORTANT NOTE: Remember, as you are reading *EAT to Your Good Health*, one of your recovery goals is to develop a positive relationship with food. Learn to appreciate all the vital nutrients that food provides, and know that your body needs these nutrients to function and feel its best. Keep in mind all the benefits that you are missing when not consuming, or digesting, a variety of healthy foods each day. Start looking at food as a positive addition to your body instead of a negative addition.

Let go of the all-or-nothing mindset. Do NOT be OBESEESED with avoiding foods that you perceive to be "unhealthy". To you "unhealthy" foods may include meat, carbohydrate, fat, or dessert. As you read *EAT to Your Good Health*, you will learn that many of these perceived "unhealthy" foods offer essential nutrients and play an important role in maintaining a healthy mind and body. Don't be mistaken. Even dessert has its role in healthy eating!

EAT
TO YOUR
GOOD HEALTH

EXCHANGES

STARCH

Foods on the Starch list contain similar amounts of carbohydrates per exchange.

Carbohydrates
Carbohydrates give you energy and are the body's main energy source. Your brain and nervous system rely on carbohydrates to function. Your body never stops running and demands lots of fuel to keep up with your daily activities. Replenish your body with healthy carbohydrates throughout the day to move towards good health.

Beans
Beans are a very healthy source of protein, carbohydrate, fiber, iron, B vitamins, potassium, and antioxidants. Beans are one of the highest food sources of antioxidants. The antioxidant levels in beans are comparable to the antioxidant levels in fruits and vegetables.

Good Health Tables: STARCH
Whole grains, beans, peas, and lentils are key sources of iron, magnesium, selenium, B vitamins, and fiber. The following table describes some of their health benefits.

Nutrient Benefits

Nutrient	Health Benefit
Iron	Helps red blood cells carry oxygen; aids in brain development and immune function; helps prevent anemia and infections
Magnesium	Aids in enzyme function; aids in nerve and muscles contraction; helps build strong bones
Selenium	Functions as an antioxidant, helps protect against heart disease; may help protect against cancer; helps cellular growth; enhances immune function
B vitamins	Helps convert food into energy; needed for proper brain function
Fiber	Helps maintain a healthy digestive tract; helps reduce risk of heart disease; may reduce risk of colon cancer

Starches, Whole grains and Phytonutrients
Many starches contain whole grains that are high in phytonutrients to help fight off disease.

Food	Phytonutrient	Health Benefit
Whole wheat	Flavonoids	Function as antioxidants; protects against cancer
Whole grains	Lignans, phytic acid	May help reduce risk of breast, colon, ovarian, and prostate cancers
Oats, potatoes	Phenolic acids	May help reduce amounts of cancer causing compounds in the body
Legumes, potatoes	Protease inhibitors	May slow tumor growth
Lentils, black-eyed peas	Tannins	Function as an antioxidant; may help reduce risk of cancer

Insufficient carbohydrate intake may lead to:
- Fatigue
- Muscle cramps
- Poor mental function including depression and anxiety
- Constipation

EXCHANGES
Each "AMOUNT" equals one starch exchange.

BREAD	AMOUNT
Bagel	¼ large (1 oz)
Bread	1 slice
Bun (hamburger, hot dog)	½ (1 oz)
Chapatti (6 inches)	1
Dinner roll	1 (1 oz)
English muffin	½
Pancake (4 inches across, ¼ inch thick)	1
Pita (6 inches)	½
Tortilla; corn, flour (6 inches)	1
Tortilla (10 inches)	⅓

CEREALS	AMOUNT
Bran, flaked	½ cup
Cooked cereal: oats, oatmeal, cream of wheat, grits	½ cup
Grape nuts, granola cereals, muesli	¼ cup
Puffed cereals	1 ½ cup
Ready-to-eat cereal, unsweetened	¾ cup
Shredded wheat; spoon size (sugar coated and plain)	½ cup
Sugar frosted cereal	½ cup

RICE, PASTA AND GRAINS

	AMOUNT
Barley, cooked	½ cup
Bulgur wheat, cooked	½ cup
Couscous	½ cup
Quinoa, cooked	½ cup
Rice, white or brown, cooked	½ cup
Pasta, cooked	½ cup
Polenta, cooked	½ cup
Tabbouleh, prepared	½ cup
Wheat germ	3 Tbsp
Wild rice, cooked	½ cup

BEANS, PEAS AND LENTILS

	AMOUNT*
Baked beans	⅓ cup
Dried beans, peas, and lentils, cooked: black, black-eyed peas, garbanzo, kidney, lentils, lima, navy, pinto, refried, white	½ cup
Peas, cooked	½ cup

CRACKERS AND SNACKS

	AMOUNT
Animal Crackers	8
Chips: tortilla, potato (fat-free, baked)	15-20 (¾ oz)
Gingersnap cookies	3
Graham crackers (2 ½ inch square)	3
Matzo	¾ oz
Melba toast (about 2 inches x 4 inches)	4 slices
Oyster crackers	20
Popcorn, popped	3 cups
Pretzels	¾ oz
Rye Crisp (2 inches x 3 ½ inches)	4
Saltine-type crackers	6
Whole wheat crackers	¾ oz

*Bean, peas, and lentils are also found on the Meat substitutes list on page 32.

STARCHY VEGETABLES	AMOUNT
Corn	½ cup
Corn on cob	½ large ear (5 oz)
Mixed vegetables with peas, corn, beans or pasta	1 cup
Parsnips	½ cup
Peas	½ cup
Plantain, ripe	½ cup
Potato, baked or broiled	¼ large or 1 small (3 oz)
Potato, mashed, prepared with milk and fat	½ cup
Spaghetti sauce	½ cup
Squash (winter, acorn, butternut, pumpkin)	1 cup
Succotash	½ cup
Sweet potato	½ cup
Yam	½ cup

OTHER STARCHES WITH ADDED FAT OR SUGAR

ITEM	AMOUNT	EXCHANGE
Biscuit, 2 ½ inches	1	1 carbohydrate, 1 fat
Chow mein noodles	½ cup	1 carbohydrate, 1 fat
Crackers		
Baked cheese type	25 grams	1 carbohydrate, 1 fat
Butter type	6	1 carbohydrate, 1 fat
Sandwich-style	3	1 carbohydrate, 1 fat
Whole-wheat	2-5 (¾ oz)	1 carbohydrate, 1 fat
Chips; tortilla, potato	9-13 (¾ oz)	1 carbohydrate, 1 fat
Cornbread (1 ¾ inch cube)	1 (1 ½ oz)	1 carbohydrate, 1 fat
Croissant		
Small	1 (1.1 oz)	1 carbohydrate, 1 fat
Large	1 (3 oz)	2 ½ carbohydrates, 3 fats
Croutons	1 cup	1 carbohydrate, 1 fat
French-Fried potatoes	15-25 (3 oz)	1 carbohydrate, 1 fat
Granola	¼ cup	1 carbohydrate, 1 fat
Granola bar	1 bar	1 carbohydrate, 1 fat
Muffin, (2 oz)	½ muffin	1 carbohydrate, 1 fat
Quick bread		
Banana	1 inch slice (2 oz)	2 carbohydrates, 1 fat
Pumpkin	1 inch slice (3 oz)	2 carbohydrates, 1 fat
Zucchini	1 inch slice (3 oz)	2 carbohydrates, 1 fat
Stuffing, prepared	⅓ cup	1 carbohydrate, 1 fat
Taco shell (5 inches)	2	1 carbohydrate, 1 fat
Waffle (4 inches across)	1	1 carbohydrate, 1 fat

NOTE: 1 starch exchange is equal to 15 grams of carbohydrate. Some basic starch exchanges include; 1 slice of bread, ¾ cup of read-to-eat cereal, ⅓ cup of cooked rice, ⅓ cup of cooked pasta, ½ cup cooked cereal, ½ cup of cooked starchy vegetable, or ¾ ounces to 1 ounce of most crackers, pretzels, and chips.

Guesstimating Starch Portion Sizes
- 1 bagel is about the size of a 6 oz tuna can
- ⅓ cup pasta, rice, or potato (1 starch exchange) is about the size of a baseball
- A medium potato is about the size of a computer mouse
- 1 slice of bread or 1 pancake (1 starch exchange) is about the size of a DVD
- 1 oz snack food is about 1 open handful

OTHER CARBOHYDRATES

CONDINMENTS

ITEM	AMOUNT	EXCHANGE
Barbeque sauce	3 Tbsp	1 carbohydrate
Honey	1 Tbsp	1 carbohydrate
Jam or jelly	1 Tbsp	1 carbohydrate
Sugar	1 Tbsp	1 carbohydrate
Syrup Chocolate & pancake	2 Tbsp	2 carbohydrates

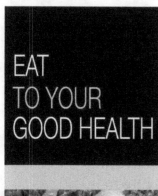

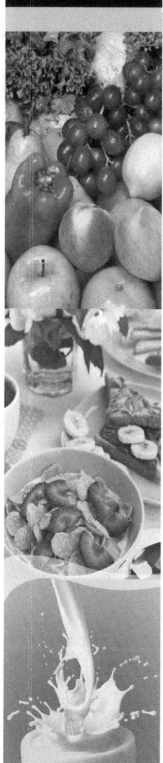

FRUITS

FRUITS

Fruits are a nutritional powerhouse. Fruits are loaded with vitamins, minerals, fiber, antioxidants, and other phytonutrients. Fruits aid in immune function, help reduce the risk of chronic disease, promote healing, and help manage weight. Consuming 5-9 servings of fruit and vegetables every day promotes good health.

Good Health Tables: FRUITS

The following table describes health benefits of some of the common nutrients found in fruit.

Nutrient Benefits

Nutrient	Health Benefit
Antioxidants	Helps protect your cells from damage; helps fight off disease
Potassium	Helps maintain a healthy blood pressure; maintains health bones; maintains cellular fluid and electrolyte balance; helps muscles contract; helps send nerve signals
Fiber	Helps maintain a healthy digestive tract; reduces risk of heart disease; may reduce risk of colon cancer
Vitamin C	Functions as an antioxidant; helps maintain a healthy immune system; helps heal cuts and bruises; important for healthy teeth and gums; aids in iron absorption
Vitamin A	Helps maintain normal vision; maintains healthy skin; regulates cell growth; maintains a healthy immune system; protects the body against infections; maintains mucous membranes
Vitamin E	Functions as an antioxidant; stabilizes cell membranes; aids in heart health
Folate	Helps form new cells; reduces risk of neural tube defects during fetal development; reduces risk of breast cancer

Fruits and Antioxidants

Fruit contains loads of antioxidants that help protect you from disease and promote good health. Additionally, antioxidants give fruit its lively color.

Color	Antioxidant	Health Benefit	Fruit
Red	Lycopene	May help reduce risk of cancer	Cherries, cranberries, guava, papaya, pink grapefruit, red grapes, strawberries, tomatoes, watermelon
Orange/Yellow	Beta-carotene	May reduce risk of heart disease and cancer; helps maintain healthy vision	Apricots, cantaloupe, carrots, papayas, yellow tomatoes
Green	Lutein (a yellow hue but masked by the plant's chlorophyll	Helps maintain healthy vision	Avocado, green apples, green grapes, honeydew, kiwi, lime, green pears
Blue/Purple	Anthocyanins	Aids in brain and immune function	Blueberries, grapes, figs, blackberries, strawberries, plums, raisins

Insufficient fruit intake may lead to:
- A compromised immune system
- Eye and skin disorders
- Vitamin and mineral deficiencies
- An increased risk of chronic disease

EXCHANGES

Each "AMOUNT" equals one fruit exchange.

FRESH FRUIT	AMOUNT*
Apple, banana, guava, kiwi, nectarine, orange, peach, tangelo	1 small-medium (4-5 oz)
Blackberries or blueberries	¾ cup
Cantaloupe or honeydew melon	1 cup cubed (11 oz)
Cherries	12 (3 oz)
Grapefruit	½ large
Grapes	17 small (3 oz)
Kumquats	5 medium
Mango	½ small or ½ cup
Papaya	½ fruit or 1 cup cubed (8 oz)
Pear	½ large (4 oz)
Persimmons	2 medium
Pineapple	¾ cup
Plum	2 small (5 oz)
Raspberries	1 cup
Strawberries	1 ¼ cup whole berries
Tangerines	2 small (8 oz)
Watermelon	1 ¼ cups cubes (13 ½ oz)

*weight includes skin, core, seeds, and rind

DRIED FRUITS	AMOUNT
Apples, dried	4 rings
Apricots, dried	8 halves
Dried fruits (berries, mixed fruits, raisins)	2 Tbsp
Figs	1 ½
Prunes	3

CANNED FRUIT	AMOUNT
Applesauce	½ cup
Fruit cocktail	½ cup
Grapefruit, canned	¾ cup
Mandarin oranges, canned	¾ cup
Peaches, canned	½ cup
Pears, canned	½ cup
Pineapple, canned	½ cup

FRUIT JUICE	AMOUNT
Apple juice/cider	½ cup
Cranberry juice cocktail	½ cup
Fruit juice blends, 100% juice	½ cup
Grape juice	½ cup
Grapefruit juice	½ cup
Nectars	½ cup
Orange juice	½ cup
Pineapple juice	½ cup
Prune juice	½ cup
Tangerine juice	½ cup

NOTE: Some basic fruit exchanges include: 1 small to medium fresh fruit, 1 cup of fresh fruit, ½ cup of canned fruit, ½ cup fruit juice, or 2 tablespoons of dried fruit.

Guesstimating Fruits Portion Sizes
- 1 cup of chopped fruit or 1 medium fresh fruit are each equal approximately the size of your fist or a tennis ball
- 2 Tbsp of dried mixed fruit or raisins (1 fruit exchange) is about the size of 1 golf ball

DAIRY

DAIRY

Milk, yogurt, and cheese are chief sources of calcium and other nutrients needed for strong bones and teeth. Osteoporosis, porous bone, is a disease that results from insufficient calcium intake. Children and adolescents are at high risk for developing osteoporosis due to the lack of calcium intake during peak bone development.

Good Health Table: MILK

Milk provides more than just calcium! The following table describes the health benefits of 9 vital nutrients that milk provides in substantial amounts. The body needs these nutrients not only for healthy bones, but also for healthy muscle and tissue function. Make sure to drink milk 3-4 times a day as a positive addition to your body.

Nutrient Benefits

Nutrient	Health Benefit
Calcium	Helps build strong bones and teeth; important for healthy nerve function, muscles contraction, and blood clotting
Protein	Builds and repairs worn out cells; needed for muscle strength and maintenance; is an energy source during intense endurance exercise
Vitamin A	Helps maintain normal vision; maintains healthy skin; regulates cell growth; maintains a healthy immune system; protects the body against infections; maintains mucous membranes
Vitamin D	Needed for calcium absorption; improves bone mineralization
Niacin	Helps convert food into energy; helps enzymes function
Riboflavin	Helps convert food into energy; helps maintain normal vision; aids in skin health
Phosphorus	Building material for bones; helps maintain bone strength; promotes energy in the body's cells
Potassium	Helps maintain a healthy blood pressure; maintains health bones; maintains cellular fluid and electrolyte balance; helps muscles contract; helps send nerve signals
Vitamin B12	Helps formation of red blood cells; maintains healthy nerve cells; used by every body cell

CALCIUM INTAKE FACTS:

Calcium Recommendations[2]

Ages	Calcium Recommendations	Dairy Amount Needed
9-18	1300 mg/day	4 servings/day
19-50	1000 mg/day	3 servings/day
51-70	1000 mg/day for male 1200 mg/day for female	3-4 servings/day

Percentage of boys and girls that do not meet their calcium recommendations[3]

Ages	Male	Female
6-11	44%	58%
12-19	64%	87%
≥ 20	55%	78%

---

[2] Committee to Review Dietary Reference Intakes for Vitamin D and Calcium Food and Nutrition Board. (2010) Dietary reference intakes for calcium and vitamin D. Institute of Medicine of the National Academies. Washington, DC: National Academy Press.

[3] Results from the United States Department of Agriculture's Continuing Survey of Food Intakes by Individuals/Diet and Health Knowledge Survey. (1994-96), as cited in National Institute of Health, Office of Dietary Supplements. (2005) *Dietary supplement fact sheet calcium*. [online] Available at: http://www.midwiferyservices.org/Calcium%20Fact%20Sheet%20NIH.pdf. [Accessed 16 June 2012].

EXCHANGES
Each "AMOUNT" equals one milk exchange.

MILK*	AMOUNT
Acidophilus Milk, Kefir	1 cup
Buttermilk	1 cup
Flavored milk (chocolate, strawberry)**	1 cup
Goat's milk	1 cup
Lactaid	1 cup
Milk (fat-free, 1%, 2%, whole)	1 cup

MILK PRODUCTS	AMOUNT
Dry Milk Powder	⅓ cup
Evaporated milk	½ cup
Yogurt***	⅔ cup (6 oz)

CHEESE****	AMOUNT*****
Cheese, Natural	1 oz
Cheese, Shredded	¼ cup
Sliced (Processed or Deli)	1 slice
String	1 piece

DAIRY-LIKE PRODUCTS	AMOUNT
Eggnog	½ cup
Rice drink	1 cup
Smoothies	10 oz
Soy milk	1 cup

*Coconut milk and dairy fats such as cream are found on the Fats list.

**Add 1 carbohydrate exchange

***Greek yogurts are located on the Meat, Cheese, and Meat Substitutes list due to the high protein content, page 31.

****Cheese is also located on the Meat, Cheese, and Meat Substitutes list due to their high protein content, page 31.

*****Some types of cheese contain less calcium than milk and yogurt. Be aware that eating cheese for your dairy choice may not meet your daily calcium recommendation. Choose milk and yogurt most often.

NOTE: Some basic dairy exchanges include: 1 cup milk, 2/3 cup (6 oz) of yogurt, and 1 oz of cheese.

Guesstimating Dairy Portion Sizes

- 1 oz of natural cheese (1 dairy exchange) is about the size of 4 game dice
- 1 cup of milk (1 dairy exchange) is about the size of your fist

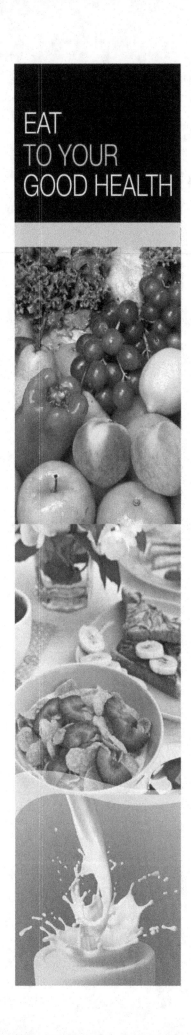

EAT
TO YOUR
GOOD HEALTH

NONSTARCHY
VEGETABLES

NONSTARCHY VEGETABLES

Vegetables, similar to fruits, also are a nutritionally dense source of vitamins, minerals, fiber, antioxidants, and other phytonutrients. Consuming 5-9 servings of fruit and vegetables every day promotes good health.

Good Health Tables: NONSTARCHY VEGETABLES

The following tables describe the main health benefits of some of the common nutrients nonstarchy vegetables provide.

Nutrient Benefits

Nutrient	Health Benefit
Antioxidants	Helps protect your cells from damage
Potassium	Helps maintain a healthy blood pressure; healthy bones; cellular fluid and electrolyte balance; helps muscles contract; helps send nerve signals
Fiber	Helps maintain a healthy digestive tract; reduce risk of heart disease; may reduce risk of colon cancer
Vitamin A	Helps maintain normal vision; maintains healthy skin; regulates cell growth; maintains a healthy immune system; protects the body against infections; maintains mucous membranes
Vitamin C	Functions as an antioxidant; helps maintain a healthy immune system; heals cuts and bruises; important for healthy teeth and gums; aids in iron absorption
Folate	Helps form new cells; reduces risk of neural tube defects during fetal development; reduces risk of breast cancer
Indoles	A group of phytonutrients found in cruciferous vegetables (flowering vegetables whose four petals resemble a cross) such as broccoli, cauliflower, and cabbage that help protect against cancer

Vegetables and Antioxidants
Vegetables contain thousands of antioxidants and phytochemicals that help protect you from disease and promote optimal health. Many antioxidants are listed below.

Color	Antioxidant	Health Benefit	Vegetable
Red	Lycopene	May reduce risk of cancer	Beets, red onions, red potatoes, rhubarb, tomatoes
Orange/ Yellow	Beta-carotene	May reduce risk of heart disease and cancer; helps maintain healthy vision	Sweet potatoes, pumpkins, carrots, butternut squash, yellow peppers, corn, yellow tomatoes, yellow beets
Green	Lutein (a yellow hue but masked by the plant's chlorophyll	Helps maintain healthy vision	Dark leafy greens, green beans, okra, green peppers, peas, cucumber, celery
Blue/ Purple	Anthocyanins	Aids in brain and immune function	Eggplant, purple onion, purple potatoes, purple cabbage
White/ Brown	Allicin	Helps lower cholesterol and blood pressure	Cauliflower, garlic, ginger, jicama, mushrooms, onions, parsnips, potatoes, turnips

Insufficient nonstarchy vegetable intake leads to:
Poor intake of important vitamins, minerals, antioxidants, phytonutrients, and fiber that help reduce the risk of chronic disease such as obesity, heart disease, and cancer.

EXCHANGES

NONSTARCHY VEGETBLES

Artichoke	Gourds	Radishes
Asparagus	Green beans	Rutabaga
Baby corn	Green onions/scallions	Salad greens
Bamboo shoots	Hearts of palm	Sauerkraut
Bean sprouts	Jicama	Snow peas
Beets	Leeks	Sprouts
Bok choy	Lettuce	Squash (summer,
Broccoli	Mixed vegetables (without	crookneck, zucchini)
Brussels sprouts	corn, peas, beans, or pasta)	Sugar snap peas
Cabbage	Mushrooms	Tomato
Carrots	Okra	Tomatoes sauce
Cauliflower	Onions	Turnips
Celery	Pea pods	Water chestnuts
Cucumber	Peppers (all varieties	Wax beans
Eggplant		

NOTE: Some vegetables contain carbohydrates and therefore are located on the Starch list. These starchy vegetables include; corn, peas, potatoes, winter squash, beans, and lentils.

Some basic nonstarchy vegetable exchanges include; ½ cup of cooked vegetables, ½ cup of vegetable juice, 1 cup raw vegetables, and 2 cups salad greens.

Guesstimating Non-starchy Vegetable Portion Sizes
- ½ cup of cooked vegetable (1 vegetable exchange) is about the size of a light bulb
- 1 cup of raw vegetable is about the size of your fist

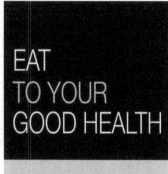

EAT
TO YOUR
GOOD HEALTH

MEAT, CHEESE and
MEAT SUBSTITUTES

MEAT, CHEESE and MEAT SUBSTITUTES

Meat, cheese, and meat substitutes provide substantial amounts of protein. Every cell in your body contains protein. Protein is needed for:

- Growth, repair, and maintenance of body tissue and cells
- Enzymes that are used for chemical reactions
- Hormones
- Immune function
- Energy
- Transportation of substances
- Blood clotting
- Structural maintenance for skin, tendons, muscles, organs, bones, and ligaments
- Prevention of chronic disease
- Promotion of optimal health

IMPORTANT NOTE: Some protein choices such as herring, mackerel, salmon, sardines, halibut, trout, and tuna are rich in omega- 3 fats, which are beneficial in heart disease.

Good health table: MEAT

The following table describes additional health benefits of the common nutrients that the Meat, Plant-Based Proteins, and Cheese group provide.

Nutrient Benefits

Nutrient	Food	Health Benefit
Iron	Beef	Help red blood cells carry oxygen; aids in brain development and immune function; helps prevent anemia and infections
Zinc	Beef, pork, poultry, shellfish	Helps enzymes function; aids in cellular growth repair; immune function; prevents birth defects during pregnancy
Thiamin	Pork, salmon	Helps convert food into energy; maintains a normal appetite; maintains nerve function
Riboflavin	Beef, pork	Helps convert food into energy; maintains normal vision; aids in skin health
Niacin	Beef, pork, poultry, fish, eggs	Helps convert food into energy; helps enzymes function

Nutrient Benefits of Meat (continued)

Nutrient	Food	Health Benefit
Vitamin B12	Beef, pork, fish	Helps formation of red blood cells; helps maintain healthy nerve cells; used by every body cell
Vitamin B6	Beef, pork, poultry, fish	Important for heart health; used for fat and protein metabolism; helps maintain healthy immune function; helps fight depression
Selenium	Beef	Functions as an antioxidant, helps protect against heart disease; may help protect against cancer; helps cellular growth; enhances immune function
Omega-3 fatty acids	Fish	Beneficial for heart health

Insufficient protein intake may lead to:
- Weakened and wasted muscles including the heart
- Impaired brain development
- Impaired thinking and learning
- Depressed metabolism
- Subnormal body temperature
- Fluid imbalance
- Electrolyte imbalance

EXCHANGES

Each "AMOUNT" equals one protein exchange.

MEATS	AMOUNT*
Bacon	
Pork	2 slices
Turkey	3 slices
Beef, chicken, game, lamb, pork, seafood, or turkey	1 oz
Beef jerky	½ oz
Cheese, natural	1 oz
Shredded	¼ cup
Sliced (processed or deli)	1 slice
String	1 piece
Cottage cheese	¼ cup
Egg	1
Ground meats	1 oz
Hot dog: single meat or combination	1
Luncheon meats	1 oz
Organ meats	1 oz
Oysters, fresh or frozen	6 medium
Ricotta cheese	¼ cup
Sardines, canned	2 small
Yogurt, Greek	3 oz

*cooked weight after bone and fat have been removed

PLANT-BASED PROTEINS* AMOUNT   EXCHANGE

PLANT-BASED PROTEINS*	AMOUNT	EXCHANGE
Baked beans	⅓ cup	1 starch, 1 protein
Dry beans, peas, and lentils, cooked: black, black-eyed peas, garbanzo, kidney, lentils, lima, navy, pinto, refried, split, white**	½ cup	1 starch, 1 protein
Edamame	½ cup	½ starch, 1 protein
Hummus	½ cup	1 starch, 1 protein
Peanut butter***	1 ½ Tbsp	1 protein
Soy-based		
Bacon	3 strips	1 protein
Burger	3 oz	½ starch, 2 proteins
Crumbles	2 oz	½ starch, 1 protein
Hot dog	1 (1 ½ oz)	½ starch, 1 protein
Nuggets	2 nuggets (1 ½ oz)	½ starch, 1 protein
Sausage patties	1 (1 ½ oz)	1 protein
Soy nuts	¾ oz	½ starch, 1 protein
Tempeh	¼ cup	1 protein
Tofu	4 oz (½ cup)	1 protein

*May also count as a carbohydrate choice
** Beans, peas, and lentils are also located on the Starch list, page 10
*** Peanut butter is also located on the Fats list, page 36

NOTE: A basic protein exchange is 1 oz of meat or cheese. 6-7 grams of protein equals 1 protein exchange.

Meat and Meat Substitutes' Portion Sizes
- 1 oz of cooked meat (1 protein exchange) is about the size of a matchbox
- 3 oz of cooked meat (3 protein exchanges) is about the size of a deck of cards or a computer mouse
- 3 oz of cooked fish (3 protein exchanges) is about the size of a checkbook
- 1 Tbsp of peanut butter (1 protein exchange) is about the size of your thumb tip
- 1 oz of natural cheese (1 protein exchange) is about the size of 4 game dice

FATS

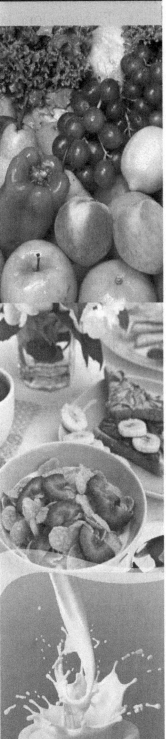

EAT
TO YOUR
GOOD HEALTH

FATS

Your body needs dietary fat every day to function properly. Eating fat does not necessarily make you fat. Maintaining a fat-free or very low fat diet is unhealthy and can lead to severe health consequences. Nutrition experts want you to understand that fat is not evil.

Benefits of dietary fat and body fat include:
- Provides long lasting energy
- Fuels muscular work
- Protects organs against shock
- Insulates the body and helps regulate body temperature
- Forms the cell membrane on all body cells
- Is converted to other compounds such as hormones and vitamin D
- Provides essential fatty acids beneficial for heart health
- Provide a dense source of energy
- Provides transportation and absorption for fat-soluble vitamins A, D, E, and K
- Helps regulate hunger and satiety signals
- Contributes to taste, smell, and texture of food

The human body is designed to have fat on it because it needs fat to survive. Stop fighting nature and accept your body.

Good Health Table: FATS
The following table describes the main health benefits of fat and some of the common nutrients that the fat group provides.

Nutrient Benefits

Food	Health Benefit
Avocado	May reduce risk of heart disease, high in healthy fats, antioxidants, vitamins and minerals
Olives	May reduce risk of heart disease, high in healthy fats, antioxidants, vitamins and minerals
Nuts	May reduce risk of heart disease, high in healthy fats, high in antioxidants, high in vitamins and minerals
Vitamin E	Functions as an antioxidant; helps stabilize cell membranes; aids in heart health

Nutrient Benefits of Fats (continued)

Food	Health Benefit
Vitamin A	Helps maintain normal vision; maintains healthy skin; regulates cell growth; maintains a healthy immune system; protect the body against infections; maintains mucous membranes
Flaxseed	High in the phytonutrients, lignans, which may help reduce risk of breast, colon, ovarian, and prostate cancers

Insufficient fat intake results in:
- Kidney disorders
- Liver disorders
- Skin abnormalities
- Signs of reproductive failure
- Fatigue
- Poor mental function
- Skin problems
- Poor wound healing
- Vitamin and mineral deficiencies due to inadequate absorption of fat-soluble vitamins

Some types of fat are healthier than other types of fat. The healthier fats, unsaturated fats, are monounsaturated and polyunsaturated fats. Monounsaturated fats such as avocado, nuts, and olive oil are derived from plant sources, while polyunsaturated fats such as nuts, salmon, and tuna are derived from plant sources and fish. Unsaturated fats are known to be heart healthy.

Saturated and *trans* fats are found in animal products such as beef and cheese; baked goods such as cookies and pastries; and many fried foods such as fried chicken and French fries. Excessive saturated and *trans* fat intake has been linked to increased risk of heart disease and high blood pressure.

Remember: Nutrition experts do not recommend avoiding fat or eating only a very small amount of fat. This approach is dangerous both physically and mentally. Do not label fat as "bad" or label foods that contain fat as "bad". You body needs fat to be at its healthiest.

EXCHANGES
Each "AMOUNT" equals one fat exchange.

FATS	AMOUNT
Avocado	2 Tbsp
Bacon, cooked, regular or turkey	1 slice
Butter, margarine, mayonnaise, or oil	1 tsp
Butter blends made with oil, regular	1 Tbsp
Coconut	
Milk	1 ½ Tbsp
Shredded	2 Tbsp
Cream	
Half and half	2 Tbsp
Heavy	1 Tbsp
Whipped	2 Tbsp
Whipped, pressurized	¼ cup
Cream cheese	1 Tbsp
Hummus	4 Tbsp
Lard	1 tsp
Mayonnaise-style salad dressing	2 tsp
Nuts	⅛ cup
Olives	
Black	8 large
Green	10 large
Peanut butter (smooth or crunchy)	½ Tbsp
Salad dressing	
Reduced-fat	2 Tbsp
Regular	1 Tbsp
Seeds	1 Tbsp
Shortening	1 tsp
Sour cream	2 Tbsp
Tahini or sesame paste	2 tsp

NOTE: A basic fat exchange is equal to 5 grams of fat.

Guesstimating Fats Portion Sizes
- 1 tsp of oil (1 fat exchange) is about the size of a quarter
- 2 Tbsp of salad dressing (2 fat exchanges) is about the size of a ping-pong ball
- 1 tsp of butter (1 fat exchange) is about the size of your fingertip

FREE FOODS

FREE FOODS

ITEMS

Bouillon	Relish
Cocktail sauce	Pickles (dill, sweet)
Ketchup or steak sauce	Salsa
Garlic	Soy sauce
Herbs and spices	Sweet chili sauce
Horseradish	Taco sauce
Hot sauce	Unsweetened beverages
Lemon juice	Vinegar
Miso	Worcestershire sauce
Mustard	

Many foods do not fit into the previous exchange categories. When these foods are consumed in reasonable amounts they do not get counted towards your daily caloric intake.

COMBINATION
FOODS

COMBINATION FOODS

ENTREES	AMOUNT	EXCHANGE
Burrito (beef and bean)	1 (8 oz)	3 carbohydrates, 3 proteins, 3 fats
Casseroles: beef or tuna noodle, lasagna, spaghetti with meat sauce or meatballs, macaroni and cheese	1 cup (8 oz)	2 carbohydrates, 2 proteins
Pot pie	1 (7 oz)	2 ½ carbohydrates, 1 protein, 3 fats
Stews (meat and vegetable)	1 cup (8 oz)	1 carbohydrate, 1 protein, 0-3 fats

SASHIMI/SUSHI	AMOUNT	EXCHANGE
Sashimi (1 piece fish over rice)	1 piece	½ carbohydrate, 1 protein
Sushi		
California roll	1 roll (6-8 pcs)	2 ½ carbohydrates, 1 protein, ½ fat
Salmon, tuna, or yellowtail roll	1 roll (6-8 pcs)	2 carbohydrates, 1 protein
Vegetable roll	1 roll (6-8 pcs)	2 carbohydrates

SALADS	AMOUNT	EXCHANGE
Coleslaw	½ cup	1 carbohydrate, 1 ½ fats
Pasta salad	½ cup	2 carbohydrates, 3 fats
Potato salad	½ cup	2 carbohydrates, 1-2 fats
Tuna or chicken salad	½ cup (3 ½ oz)	½ carbohydrate, 2 proteins, 1 fat

FAST FOODS

FAST FOODS

PIZZA	AMOUNT	EXCHANGE
Cheese, thin crust	¼ of a 12 inch (about 6 oz)	2 ½ carbohydrates, 1 protein, 1 ½ fats
Meat, regular crust	1/8 of a 14 inch (about 4 oz)	2 ½ carbohydrates, 2 proteins, 1 ½ fats

FOOD	AMOUNT	EXCHANGE
Asian (beef, chicken, or shrimp) with vegetables in sauce	1 cup	1 carbohydrate, 1 protein, 1 fat
Asian noodles with vegetables in sauce	1 cup	2 carbohydrates, 1 fat
Chicken sandwich, grilled	1	3 carbohydrates, 4 proteins
Chicken sandwich, fried	1	3 ½ carbohydrates, 3 proteins, 1 fat
French fries	Small	3 carbohydrates, 3 fats
	Medium	4 carbohydrates, 4 fats
	Large	5 carbohydrates, 6 fats
Hamburger Large with cheese	1	2 ½ carbohydrates, 4 proteins, 1 fat
Regular (kid size)	1	2 carbohydrates, 1 protein, 1 fat
Onion rings	About 3 oz (4-5 rings)	2 ½ carbohydrates, 3 fats
Submarine sandwich	6-inch sub	3 carbohydrates, 2 proteins, 1 fat
Taco, hard or soft shell (meat and cheese)	1 small	1 carbohydrate, 1 protein, 1 ½ fats

FOOD IS GOOD

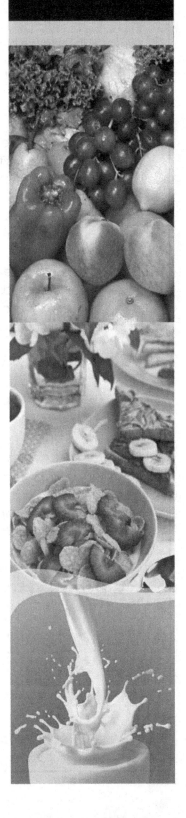

EAT
TO YOUR
GOOD HEALTH

FOOD IS GOOD

WHY YOU SHOULD EAT HAMBURGERS & BURRITOS:

Yes, I said it; there are benefits to burgers and burritos. It's possible to get health benefits from some comfort foods. Play around and get creative with adding nutrient rich toppings. You can have your burger or burrito and eat it too!

Hamburger with toppings:

- A whole wheat bun provides:
  - Fiber to promote regularity, heart health, and a reduced risk of cancer
  - Phytochemicals to promote a reduced risk of cancer
  - Carbohydrates for energy
- Mushrooms, onions, and dark leafy greens provide:
  - Phytochemicals to promote immune health and a reduced risk of cancer
  - Fiber to promote regularity, heart health, and a reduced risk of cancer
- Avocado provides:
  - Monounsaturated fat to promote heart health
  - Antioxidants, vitamins, minerals, and fiber to promote immune health, heart health, and a reduced risk of cancer
- Ketchup and a tomato slice provides vitamins and lycopene to promote a reduced risk of cancer
- Lean beef provides vitamins, minerals, protein, and fat needed to keep us strong and healthy

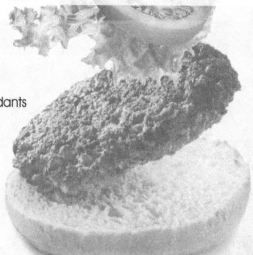

Burrito with fillings (in a briefer description):

- A tortilla provides whole grain
- Beans provide carbohydrate, protein, fiber, and antioxidants
- Onions provide phytochemicals
- Cheese provides protein, fat, and calcium
- Lean beef provides vitamins, minerals, protein, and fat
- Tomatoes provide vitamins and lycopene
- Salsa provides vitamins, minerals, and phytochemicals

MEAL PLANNING

MEAL PLANNING

FOR YOU

Your dietitian will provide you with exchanges for each meal and snack, or provide you with your total daily exchanges and let you plan your meals and snacks accordingly.

During the initial phases of treatment, it may be very difficult for you to plan your meals and snacks. In this case, your dietitian will help provide you with the proper exchanges for each meal and snack. An important part of your recovery is learning to be relaxed around food and not have rigid eating behaviors. Planning your own meals and snacks by using your recommended daily exchanges is one way to move toward relaxed eating behaviors. Keep in mind that it is best to consume balanced meals that include food from all food groups, which will provide you with adequate nutrition and help fight off food cravings.

Your meal plan will be clear and direct. This will help prevent any confusion that may allow eating disorder thoughts and behaviors to stray you from the meal plan. You are expected to consume all of the food on your plate. Do not leave any crumbs behind. Additionally, if you are complaining of fullness when you eat, than it may be better for you to drink your fruit and vegetables rather than eat them.

FOR REGISTERED DIETITIANS

Meal plans will vary among dietitians. Exchanges can be arranged in several ways to meet a single caloric goal. The calories from the following sample meal plans are listed for the dietitian's use only, and these pages should be removed prior to providing *EAT to Your Good Health* to your client. The patient's meal plan will not have the calories displayed. Each sample meal plan is based on low-fat milk and a combination of very lean, lean, and medium-fat meat types. If the patient is only choosing very lean meat options, than add 1 fat with each meal to obtain the stated calorie amount. Most meat choices for the meal plans are lean and medium-lean proteins. Furthermore, using your discretion, you may feel that it is appropriate to add foods to these exchange lists, such as select reduced fat foods and soups, on a case-by-case basis and depending on patient's recovery stage.

The exchanges may be moved around to meet a patient's likes. For example, if the patient would rather have a fruit with a snack instead of with lunch, than move the exchange accordingly. Or, if the patient would rather have a fat with the evening snack instead of breakfast, than move the fat accordingly. When incorporating dessert select a lower calorie meal plan then add dessert to that plan to reach the desired calorie goal. Dessert exchanges have been left off *EAT to Your Good Health* exchange lists. Desserts should be in addition to base nutrients and not replacement of base nutrients. Desserts are an essential part of a happy healthy meal plan.

Blank meal plan forms are located on pages 68 - 79 of this booklet. You may use these forms to provide your patient with his/her prescribed meal plans. Additional copies may be downloaded at www.beenutritious.com.

SAMPLE MEAL PLANS

1200 Calorie

Meal/Snack	Starch	Fruit	Dairy	Vegetable	Protein	Fat
Breakfast	1	1	1		1	
AM Snack						
Lunch	1	1	1		2	1
PM Snack					1	
Dinner	1		1		2	1
Evening Snack		1				
Total	3	3	3		6	2

1400 Calorie

Meal/Snack	Starch	Fruit	Dairy	Vegetable	Protein	Fat
Breakfast	1	1	1		1	1
AM Snack						
Lunch	2	1	1	0.5	2	1
PM Snack					1	
Dinner	2		1	0.5	2	1
Evening Snack		1				
Total	5	3	3	1	6	3

1600 Calorie

Meal/Snack	Starch	Fruit	Dairy	Vegetable	Protein	Fat
Breakfast	1	1	1		1	1
AM Snack						
Lunch	2	1	1	0.5	2	1
PM Snack	1				1	
Dinner	2		1	0.5	2	1
Evening Snack		1	1			
Total	6	3	4	1	6	3

SAMPLE MEAL PLANS

1800 Calorie

Meal/Snack	Starch	Fruit	Dairy	Vegetable	Protein	Fat
Breakfast	2	1	1		1	1
AM Snack						
Lunch	2	1	1	0.5	2	1
PM Snack	1				1	
Dinner	2		1	0.5	3	1
Evening Snack		1	1			
Total	7	3	4	1	7	3

2000 Calorie

Meal/Snack	Starch	Fruit	Dairy	Vegetable	Protein	Fat
Breakfast	2	1	1		1	1
AM Snack		1				
Lunch	2	1	1	0.5	3	1
PM Snack	1				1	
Dinner	2		1	0.5	4	2
Evening Snack		1	1			
Total	7	4	4	1	9	4

2200 Calorie

Meal/Snack	Starch	Fruit	Dairy	Vegetable	Protein	Fat
Breakfast	2	1	1		1	1
AM Snack		1				
Lunch	3	1	1	0.5	3	2
PM Snack	1				1	
Dinner	3		1	1	4	2
Evening Snack		1	1			
Total	9	4	4	1.5	9	5

Note: The registered dietitian should remove the "Sample Meal Plans" pages prior to providing *EAT to Your Good Health* to his/her client.

HUNGER AND SATIETY

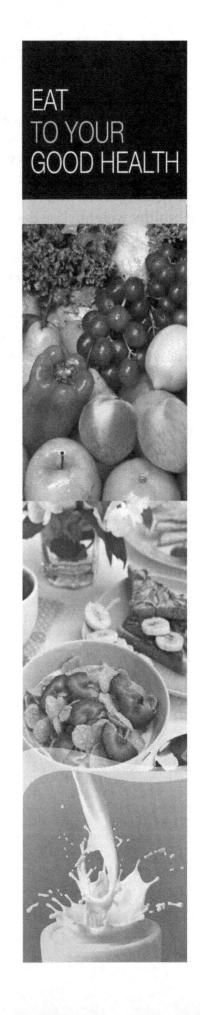

EAT
TO YOUR
GOOD HEALTH

HUNGER AND SATIETY

One of your treatment goals is to get in-touch with your body's hunger and satiety signals. Satiety is the state of being satisfied. When I talk about satiety levels I'm saying, "How satisfied are you with your meal or snack?" It is important to trust your body to provide you with the right eating cues whether the cues are barely felt or painful. Listening to your body by eating when you're hungry and stopping when you're full is a great method to maintain a healthy weight. Use the hunger and satiety scales located in this book as a tool to rate your hunger throughout the day. Think of it as "checking in" with your body to learn what it needs. It may take a little while to get your hunger and satiety signals back on track if your eating disorder behaviors disrupted them. For now, follow your meal plan whether you are hungry or not.

The huger and satiety scales are located on page 51 of this booklet. Additional copies may be downloaded at www.beenutritious.com.

HUNGER
SATIETY SCALES

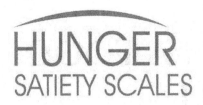
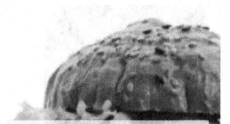

Hunger and satiety scales are a great tool to help you maintain a healthy weight. Use these scales to rate your hunger and satiety throughout the day. Learn the best times to begin eating and stop eating. Think of it as "checking in" with your body and listening to what your body needs.

0 is neutral and 5 is extremely starved or extremely full.

Hunger Scale

0	1	2	3	4	5
Neutral	Barely hungry	Getting hungrier. Almost ready to eat.	Definitely hungry. Ready to eat	Starved	Extremely starved, famished

- 0. Neutral
- 1. Barely hungry
- 2. Getting hungrier. Almost ready to eat.
- 3. Definitely hungry. Ready to eat. You should eat here.
- 4. Starved
- 5. Extremely starved. Famished.

Satiety Scale

0	1	2	3	4	5
Neutral	Hunger Going Away	Hunger is Gone	Definitely Full	Bloated, Stuffed, uncomfortable	Extremely full, Miserable

- 0. Neutral
- 1. Hunger is beginning to go away.
- 2. Hunger is gone but you could eat more. You are almost satisfied.
- 3. Definitely full. Satisfied. You should stop eating here.
- 4. Bloated, stuffed, and uncomfortable.
- 5. Extremely stuffed and miserable. Painful.

Letting your body get to the point of starving, or close to starving, will increase the risk of consuming less healthier food choices, eating too fast, overeating, and binging on your next meal. This, in turn, may increase feelings of disgust or the need to purge. It is best to eat when your hunger is at a 3 and stop when your satiety is at a 3.

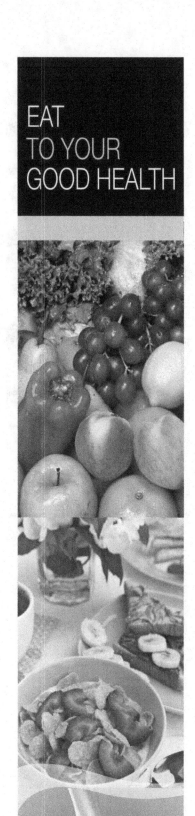

EAT
TO YOUR
GOOD HEALTH

KEEPING A FOOD JOURNAL

KEEPING A FOOD JOURNAL

Keeping a food journal is an important tool during recovery. Your food journal can help you learn how to change your eating behaviors by identifying triggers, thoughts, and behaviors. Be honest in your food journal so your treatment team can know how to best help you. Use the hunger and satiety scales for each meal and snack. Record your hunger at the start of the meal or snack, and then record your satiety once you are done eating. Be sure to record the nutrient benefits for each food consumed, which will help you become more aware of why food is such a key component of good health. Your dietitian will explain how to keep a food journal.

5 tips for keeping a food journal:
- Write food down as soon as you eat it. This may mean carrying your food journal during the day if you are on the go
- Include everything that you put in your mouth such as bites, drinks, tastes, sips, etc
- Feel free to use the other side of paper for additional foods and/or comments, or use 2 food journal forms for each day.
- Keep your personal journal separate so you can turn in your food journal
- If you copy the food journal from this booklet, than be aware that you may want it double sided for more room to write

A sample food journal is located on page 81. Blank food journal forms are located on pages 82 - 132 of this booklet. Additional copies may be downloaded at www.beenutritious.com.

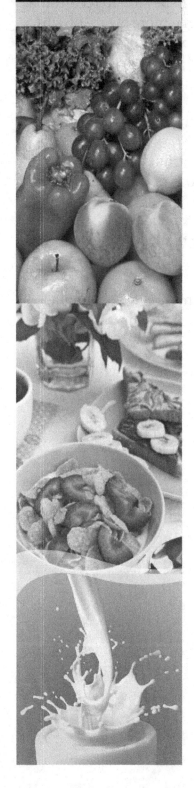

EAT
TO YOUR
GOOD HEALTH

NUTRITION CARE

NUTRITION CARE

NUTRITION MANAGEMENT

Nutrition management is not a rigid approach. It is the role of the registered dietitian to decide the best approach for each client. What is appropriate for one client may not be appropriate for another client. For example, one client may need small frequent meals, whereas another client may become overwhelmed with too many feedings and would benefit from 3 larger meals per day. Additionally, you may need to start your client on a caloric goal that is lower or higher than the following suggested initial prescription.

Anorexia Nervosa

Goals: help client establish a normal eating pattern, help client achieve a healthy body weight, and obtain medical stability.

General guidelines:

- Initial prescription in range of 1200-1400 kcal/day
- Increase prescription by 100-200 kcal every few days
- Estimate energy needs at 130% of REE
- Progress to weight gain of 1-2 pounds per week
- Encourage balanced meals
  - Carbohydrate: 50-55% of total energy
  - Fat: 25-30% of total energy
  - Protein: 15-20% of total energy[4]

Typically, I like to start my clients on a caloric meal plan that is approximately a couple hundred calories greater than the client's 3-7 day average calorie count. I feel that this approach not only helps prevent refeeding syndrome, but also creates an obtainable goal for the client.

Bulimia Nervosa

Goals: help client establish a normal eating pattern, stop binge-purge cycle (stop purging then stop binging), and stabilize body weight.

General guidelines:

- Initial prescription in range of 1200-1500 kcal/day
  - If patient's weight is stabilized, then small consistent caloric increases should be given to improve metabolic rate
- Estimate energy needs at 120-130% of REE
  - If hypometabolic estimate energy needs at 100% of REE
- Promote weight gain of 1-2 pounds per week depending on treatment type
- Encourage balanced meals
  - Carbohydrate: 50-55% of total energy
  - Fat: 25-30% of total energy
  - Protein: 15-20% of total energy[4]

---

[4] Academy of Nutrition and Dietetics. (2011 Online Edition). *Nutrition Care Manual.* Chicago, IL.

Remember to discourage dieting. One cannot diet and recover at the same time. Once the recovery process has steadily moved forward, the treatment team believes the client is doing well physically and mentally, and client has stabilized his/her weight for at least 3 months, then he/she may begin to lose weight if necessary; however, it is significant for the registered dietitian and the client to be aware that a weight-loss diet may trigger the binge/purge cycle.

NUTRITION DIAGNOSIS

Nutrition problems should be diagnosed based on the client's signs and symptoms obtained during the nutrition assessment. Some common nutrition diagnoses for anorexia nervosa and bulimia include:

- Inadequate energy intake (NI – 1.4)
- Inadequate oral intake (NI – 2.1)
- Malnutrition (NI – 5.2)
- Inadequate protein-energy intake (NI – 5.3)
- Underweight (NC – 3.1)
- Disordered eating pattern (NB – 1.5)[5]

Sample PES or Nutrition Diagnostic Statements

- Inadequate energy intake related to patient complaints that food will cause weight gain as evidenced by patient consuming approximately 650 kcal per day compared to estimated requirement of 1650 kcal per day.
- Inadequate energy intake related to disordered eating pattern and self-limiting behavior as evidenced by patient consuming approximately 650 kcal per day compared to estimated requirement of 1650 kcal per day.
- Inadequate energy intake related to the desire to be thin as evidenced by self-restricted intake of 650 kcal per day as compared to estimated requirement of 1650 kcal per day.
- Inadequate protein-energy intake related to food- and nutrition-related knowledge deficit as evidenced by omission of dietary meat due to perception that meat causes weight gain.
- Malnutrition related to intentional food restriction for weight loss as evidenced by BMI of 14 and unwillingness to eat sufficient energy/protein to maintain a healthy weight.
- Underweight related to desire to be thin as evidenced by weight for age < 3rd percentile with 11% weight loss in past month.
- Underweight related to intentional food restriction for weight loss as evidenced by current weight of 34 kg compared to a minimum healthy weight of 42 kg.
- Disordered eating pattern related to feeling "fat" as evidenced by inadequate intake at meals followed by uncontrollable excessive intake at night.
- Disordered eating pattern related to desire to be thin as evidenced by inflexibility with foods selection and chronic dieting.

Note: The registered dietitian should remove the pages in the "Nutrition Care" section prior to providing *EAT to Your Good Health* to his/her client.

---

[5] Academy of Nutrition and Dietetics. (2011 Online Edition) *International Dietetics & Nutrition Terminology Reference Manual, 3rd edition*. As cited in *Nutrition Care Manual*, Chicago, IL.

EATING DISORDER RESOURCES for PATIENTS, FAMILIES & DIETITIANS

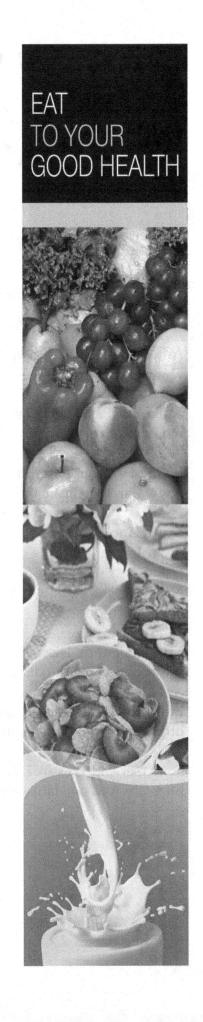

EAT
TO YOUR
GOOD HEALTH

EATING DISORDER RESOURCES for PATIENTS, FAMILIES & DIETITIANS

Academy for Eating Disorders
www.aedweb.org

American Anorexia/Bulimia Association
www.aabainc.org

American Dietetic Association
www.eatright.org

American Psychiatric Association
www.psych.org

Eating Disorder Referral and Information Center
www.edreferral.com

Gürze Books
www.bulimia.com

National Association of Anorexia Nervosa and Associated Disorders
www.anad.org

National Eating Disorders Association
www.nationaleatingdisorders.org

Educator, parent, coach, and athletic trainer toolkits available at:
http://www.nationaleatingdisorders.org/information-resources/toolkits.php

Somerset and Wessex Eating Disorders Association
http://www.swedauk.org/index.htm

READING
RECOMMENDATIONS

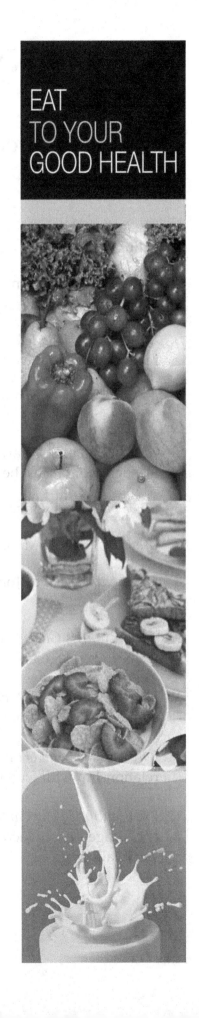

EAT
TO YOUR
GOOD HEALTH

READING RECOMMENDATIONS

Eating Disorder Books for Those in Recovery and Their Loved Ones

1. *The Rules of Normal Eating* by Karen R. Koenig describes an approach to help those with an eating disorder to get their eating under control.

2. *Life without ED* by Jenni Schaefer with Thom Rutledge is a story of how a woman freed herself from her eating disorder and how you can free yourself too.

3. *Goodby Ed, Hello Me* by Jenni Schaefer is a book that provides encouragement to help you recover from your eating disorder.

4. *Making Weight* by Arnold Andersen, Leigh Cohn , Thomas Holbrook is a men's help book about food, weight, and appearance.

5. *Next to Nothing* by Carrie Arnold with B. Timothy Walsh is an inspiring story of how a teenager almost lost her life to an eating disorder.

6. *Binge No More* by Joyce Nash is a guide to overcoming disordered eating.

7. *Crave* by Cynthia M. Bulik discusses the reasons you binge and how to stop.

8. *The Invisible Man* by John F. Morgan is a self-help guide for men with eating disorders and bigorexia.

9. *The Beginner's Guide to Eating Disorder Recovery* by Nancy Kolodny is a self-help book for teens and college-aged readers.

10. *Does This Pregnancy Make Me Look Fat?* by Claire Mysko and Magali Amadeï helps pregnant women overcome body-image challenges.

11. *Eating in the Light of the Moon* by Anita Johnston discussed how women can change their relationship with food through storytelling.

12. *I'm Beautiful? Why Can't I See It?* by Kimberly Davidson is a book that provides daily encouragement to increase self-esteem with inspirational saying including Bible study for spirituality.

13. *Self-esteem Comes in All Sizes* by Carol A. Johnson encourages you to love yourself and enjoy life no matter what your size.

14. *Feeding the Starving Mind* by Doreen A. Samuelson is a workbook that is developed for older teens and adult women with anorexia with emphasis on anxiety management.

15. *Understanding Your Loved One's Eating Disorder and How you Can Help* by Johanna Marie McShane and Tony Paulson is a book for parents and loved-ones to help understand your child's eating disorder and why she feels fat.

16. *Father Hunger* by Margo Main explains how young women develop body image and eating disorders due to physically or emotionally absent fathers.

17. *When Your Child Has an Eating Disorder* by Abigail H. Natenshon is a workbook targeted for parents who want to participate in the recovery process.

GLOSSARY

GLOSSARY

Anorexia nervosa: A type of eating disorder characterized extreme self-starvation, intense fear of being fat, and refusal to maintain a minimally normal body weight for age and height.

Antioxidant: A compound that protects the body's cells against damage. Eating antioxidants regularly can help improve immune function, repair damaged cells, and reduce risk of chronic diseases.

Binge eating disorder: A type of eating disorder characterized by recurrent episodes of binge eating without inappropriate compensatory behaviors such as purging, laxative abuse, fasting, and/or excessive exercise.

Body Mass Index: An indicator of body fat used to define a healthy weight. Generally speaking, BMI (body mass index) is calculated by dividing weight by height.

Bulimia nervosa: A type of eating disorder characterized by recurrent episodes of binge eating following by one or more inappropriate compensatory behaviors such as purging, laxative abuse, fasting, and/or excessive exercise.

Calorie: A unit of energy. A calorie is a measure of the amount of energy in food such as feet is a measure of length. You must eat food to get enough calories, or energy, for your body to function properly and stay healthy. You get calories through eating protein, carbohydrate, and fat. Protein, carbohydrate, and fat not only provide the essential calories your body needs, but they also provide you with a vast array of other important nutrients including vitamins, mineral, and antioxidants.

Carbohydrate: Compounds composed of one or more sugars including; starch, sugar, and fiber. Grains, rice, wheat, corn, potatoes, and sugar are typical sources of carbohydrate. Carbohydrates are broken down into sugar in your body, which supplies your body with energy. Carbohydrates are the body's main source of energy.

Cholesterol: A waxy substance produced by the body or found in animal foods. Cholesterol is used by your body for many necessary functions; however, too much cholesterol in the blood is associated with an increased risk of heart disease.

Chronic disease: A long-standing illness such as obesity, heart disease, cancer, and osteoporosis.

Dietary fiber: An indigestible compound that helps lower cholesterol and is beneficial for digestive health. Additionally, a lack of fiber may lead to constipation.

Eating Disorder: A condition in which poor eating behaviors compromises a person's health. Some types of eating disorders include anorexia nervosa, bulimia nervosa, and binge eating disorder.

Exchange: Similar caloric equivalents of foods within a food grouping.

Fat: A nutrient that provides long-lasting energy. The different types of fat include:

- **Omega-3 fat:** A polyunsaturated fat known for its benefit in heart heath. Omega-3 fatty acids are found in certain oils, nuts, seeds, and fish. Fatty fish such as salmon, tuna, trout, and mackerel are top sources.
- **Monounsaturated fat:** An unsaturated fat that may help reduce the risk of heart disease and help maintain a healthy blood cholesterol level. Olive oil, olives, avocado, peanut butter, and tree nuts are good sources.
- **Polyunsaturated fat:** An unsaturated fat that may help reduce risk of heart disease; aid in mental and visual health; promote healthy immune function; and support a favorable body composition. Good sources include fish (salmon, tuna, and other fish oils), beef, lamb and some cheese.
- **Saturated fat:** A fat that is typically solid at room temperature and may increase unhealthy blood cholesterol levels and arterial plaque build-up. Animal products (milk, cheese, meat fat, lard, butter), with the exception of fish, are typically rich sources of saturated fat.
- *Trans* **fatty acids:** A type of fat that occurs naturally or is man-made. The man-made type is a solid fat and adversely affects blood cholesterol levels more than saturated fat. Baked goods, tub margarines, and fried foods can be rich sources of *trans* fat.

Food groups: Foods grouped together due to their common nutrients. The five food groups include; grains, fruits, vegetables, dairy, meat and beans, and sometimes oils although technically oils is not a food group.

Malnutrition: A condition cause by nutrient or energy imbalance that can lead to serious health problems. People with eating disorders are at an increased risk of malnutrition.

Metabolic rate: The amount of energy needed, or used, to maintain your body's daily functions. If you have a high metabolic rate, or metabolism, than you burn more calories than if you had a slow metabolism. Adverse eating behaviors such as skipping meals, binging, purging, and eating too few calories can lead to a slow metabolism. Be sure to keep your body fueled throughout the day to keep your metabolism working efficiently.

Minerals: Naturally growing inorganic substances. Examples include iron, selenium, calcium, zinc, and phosphorus.

Nutrients: Carbohydrate, protein, fat, vitamins, minerals, and water, which are necessary to the body's proper functioning, are nutrients.

Osteoporosis: A condition in which bones become porous and fragile. Not consuming enough calcium and vitamin D may lead to osteoporosis. Osteoporosis is commonly found in people with eating disorders.

Phytonutrients: Plant compounds that help protect the eater against disease. *Phyto* means plant, and nutrient is a compound.

Protein: A nutrient used by the body for growth, repair, and energy. Milk, cheese, beans, meat, and soy are key sources of protein.

Registered dietitian: A dietitian with a degree in dietetics whom completed an approved internship program, passed the *registration* exam, and maintains the minimum amount of continuing education credits.

Starch: A sugar molecule from a plant source. A starch is a type of carbohydrate.

Vitamins: Organic compounds necessary for bodily functions.

REFERENCES

REFERENCES

Christie, C. Editor in Chief. (2009 Online Edition). Florida Manual of Medical Nutrition Therapy. Florida Dietetic Association, Tallahassee, FL.

Duff, R.L. (2002) 2006. *American Dietetic Association complete food and nutrition guide*. Hoboken, NJ: John Wiley & Sons, Inc.

Hart, S., Russell, J. and Abraham, S. (2011). Nutrition and dietetic practice in eating disorder management. *Journal of Human Nutrition and Dietetics* 24(2), 144-153.

Katzman, D.K. (2005). Medical complications in adolescents with anorexia nervosa: a review of the literature. *International Journal of Eating Disorders* 37, S52-S59.

Klausner, A. (2004). From avocados to yogurt: 15 super foods for super health. *Environmental Nutrition* S-1.

Mahan, K.L., Escott-Stump, S. and Raymond, J.L. (1952) 2011. *Krause's food and the nutrition care process*. Philadelphia, PA: W.B. Saunders Company.

Mathieu, J. (2009). What should you know about mindful and intuitive eating?. *Journal of the Academy of Nutrition and Dietetics* 109(12), 1982-1987.

Mehler, P.S. (2011). Medial complications of bulimia nervosa and their treatments. *International Journal of Eating Disorders* 44(2), 95-104.

National Association of Anorexia Nervosa and Associated Disorders.
    http://www.anad.org/

Sizer, F. and Whitney, E. (1980) 2011. *Nutrition: concepts and controversies*. Belmont, CA: Wadsworth, Cengage Learning.

Venes, D. (1940) 2009. *Taber's Cyclopedic medical dictionary*. Philadelphia, PA: F.A. Davis Company.

Wolfe, R. (2006). The underappreciated role of muscle in health and disease. *American Journal of Clinical Nutrition* 84(3): 475-82.

Wu, X., Beecher, G.R., Holden, J.M., Haytowitz, D.B., Gebhardt, S.E., and Prior, R.L. (2004). Lipophilic and hydrophilic antioxidant capacities of common foods in the United States. *Journal of Agricultural and Food Chemistry* 52(12), 4026-4037.

NOTES

HOW to ORDER MORE COPIES of *EAT to YOUR GOOD HEALTH*

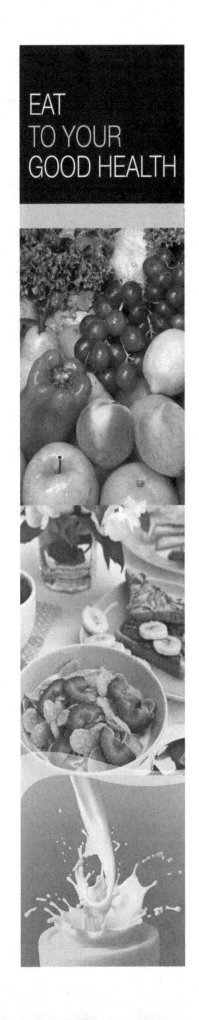

HOW TO ORDER MORE COPIES OF
EAT to Your Good Health

Please use your preferred method.

1. Order online from www.beenutritious.com
2. Email your order: a.galena@beenutritious.com
3. Call to order: 904-866-2393
4. Order through Barnes & Noble or other online retailers

BLANK MEAL PLANS

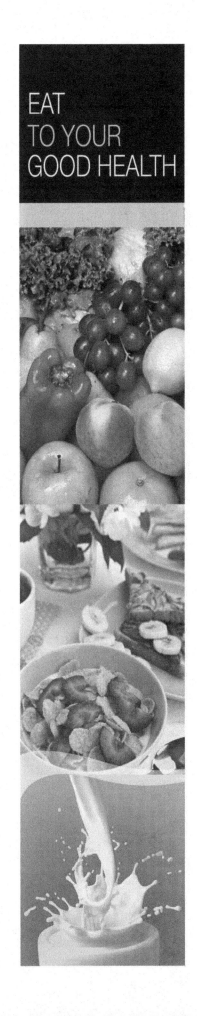

EAT
TO YOUR
GOOD HEALTH

My MEAL Plan

Name: _____

Dietitian: _____

Date [ ]

Recommended Exchanges:

Starch	Fruit	Dairy	Vegetable	Protein	Fat

Meal/Snack	Starch	Fruit	Dairy	Vegetable	Protein	Fat	Sample Menu Option	Sample Menu Option
Breakfast								
AM Snack								
Lunch								
PM Snack								
Dinner								
Evening Snack								

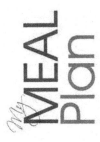

My MEAL Plan

Name:

Dietitian:

Date

Recommended Exchanges:

Starch	Fruit	Dairy	Vegetable	Protein	Fat

Meal/ Snack	Starch	Fruit	Dairy	Vegetable	Protein	Fat	Sample Menu Option	Sample Menu Option
Breakfast								
AM Snack								
Lunch								
PM Snack								
Dinner								
Evening Snack								

My MEAL Plan

Name: _____

Dietitian: _____

Date [_____]

Recommended Exchanges:

Starch	Fruit	Dairy	Vegetable	Protein	Fat

Meal/ Snack	Starch	Fruit	Dairy	Vegetable	Protein	Fat	Sample Menu Option	Sample Menu Option
Breakfast								
AM Snack								
Lunch								
PM Snack								
Dinner								
Evening Snack								

My MEAL Plan

Name: _____

Dietitian: _____

Date [_____]

Recommended Exchanges:

Starch	Fruit	Dairy	Vegetable	Protein	Fat

Meal/ Snack	Starch	Fruit	Dairy	Vegetable	Protein	Fat	Sample Menu Option	Sample Menu Option
Breakfast								
AM Snack								
Lunch								
PM Snack								
Dinner								
Evening Snack								

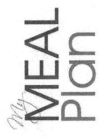

My MEAL Plan

Name: _____

Dietitian: _____

Recommended Exchanges:

Starch	Fruit	Dairy	Vegetable	Protein	Fat

Date: [   ]

Meal/Snack	Starch	Fruit	Dairy	Vegetable	Protein	Fat	Sample Menu Option	Sample Menu Option
Breakfast								
AM Snack								
Lunch								
PM Snack								
Dinner								
Evening Snack								

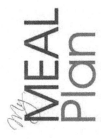

My MEAL Plan

Name: _____

Dietitian: _____

Date [_____]

Recommended Exchanges:

Starch	Fruit	Dairy	Vegetable	Protein	Fat

Meal/ Snack	Starch	Fruit	Dairy	Vegetable	Protein	Fat	Sample Menu Option	Sample Menu Option
Breakfast								
AM Snack								
Lunch								
PM Snack								
Dinner								
Evening Snack								

My MEAL Plan

Name: _____

Dietitian: _____

Date ☐

Recommended Exchanges:

Starch	Fruit	Dairy	Vegetable	Protein	Fat

Meal/ Snack	Starch	Fruit	Dairy	Vegetable	Protein	Fat	Sample Menu Option	Sample Menu Option
Breakfast								
AM Snack								
Lunch								
PM Snack								
Dinner								
Evening Snack								

My MEAL Plan

Name: _____

Dietitian: _____

Date [ ]

Recommended Exchanges:

Starch	Fruit	Dairy	Vegetable	Protein	Fat

Meal/Snack	Starch	Fruit	Dairy	Vegetable	Protein	Fat	Sample Menu Option	Sample Menu Option
Breakfast								
AM Snack								
Lunch								
PM Snack								
Dinner								
Evening Snack								

My MEAL Plan

Name: _____

Dietitian: _____

Date [   ]

Recommended Exchanges:

Starch	Fruit	Dairy	Vegetable	Protein	Fat

Meal/ Snack	Starch	Fruit	Dairy	Vegetable	Protein	Fat	Sample Menu Option	Sample Menu Option
Breakfast								
AM Snack								
Lunch								
PM Snack								
Dinner								
Evening Snack								

My MEAL Plan

Name:

Dietitian:

Date _____

Recommended Exchanges:

Starch	Fruit	Dairy	Vegetable	Protein	Fat

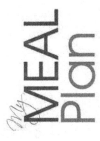

Meal/Snack	Starch	Fruit	Dairy	Vegetable	Protein	Fat	Sample Menu Option	Sample Menu Option
Breakfast								
AM Snack								
Lunch								
PM Snack								
Dinner								
Evening Snack								

My MEAL Plan

Name: _____

Dietitian: _____

Recommended Exchanges:

Starch	Fruit	Dairy	Vegetable	Protein	Fat

Date [_____]

Meal/Snack	Starch	Fruit	Dairy	Vegetable	Protein	Fat	Sample Menu Option	Sample Menu Option
Breakfast								
AM Snack								
Lunch								
PM Snack								
Dinner								
Evening Snack								

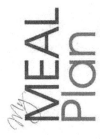

My MEAL Plan

Name: _____

Dietitian: _____

Recommended Exchanges:

Starch	Fruit	Dairy	Vegetable	Protein	Fat

Date _____

Meal/Snack	Starch	Fruit	Dairy	Vegetable	Protein	Fat	Sample Menu Option	Sample Menu Option
Breakfast								
AM Snack								
Lunch								
PM Snack								
Dinner								
Evening Snack								

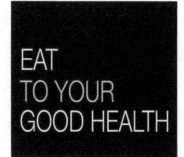

EAT
TO YOUR
GOOD HEALTH

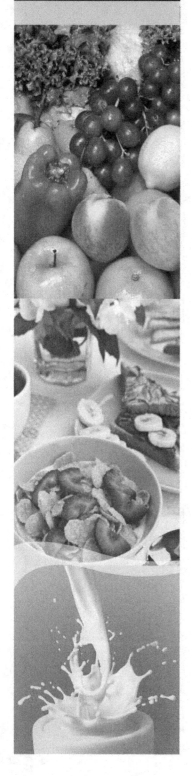

SAMPLE FOOD JOURNAL & BLANK FOOD JOURNALS

My Food Journal

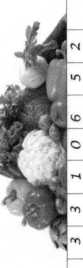

Name: Amy

Date/Day: Monday   Daily Goal(s): *stay positive / follow meal plan / be honest*

Recommended Exchanges/Consumed exchanges

Starch	Fruit	Dairy	Vegetable	Protein	Fat
5 5	3 2	3 3	1 0	6 5	2 2

Time	Food and Amount	Exchange						Hunger Scale	Nutrient Benefits	Thoughts/Feelings	Behavior
		S	F	D	V	P	F				
630	3/4 cup Cherrios	1						2, 3	grains give me energy	didn't want to eat	mean
	1 cup 2% milk			1					milk provides vit/min	followed meal plan	cried
	1 hard boiled egg					1			protein helps my muscles	feel fat	ate
	1 sm banana		1						fiber & antioxidants	sad	
1100	2 sl bread	2						3, 3	fiber for digestion	happy to get help	calm
	6 sl turkey					3			protein helps me grow strong	feel full	made myself
	1 sl cheese					1			contains protein & calcium	too much food	eat
	1 kiwi		1						helps me from getting sick	yummy	
	1 tbsp mayo						1		needed to absorb vitamins	want to hide the food	hid food
	6 oz reg yogurt			1					calcium for stong bones & teeth		
1000	8 donuts							5, 5		disgusted	binged
										ate 1 so mind as well	purged
										finish box	
										will make me fat	
										Note: the above are different examples of thoughts/feelings that you may have. Several different examples are given for each meal.	
Total		3	2	2	0	5	1				

Exercise: *walked 20 min*

Met goal: yes/**no**/improving

Met all exchanges: yes/**no**

Exchanges to make up:
1 pro, 1 fruit, 1 veg

My Food Journal

Name:

Date/Day: Daily Goal(s):

Recommended Exchanges/Consumed exchanges

Starch	Fruit	Dairy	Vegetable	Protein	Fat

Time	Food and Amount	Exchange						Hunger Scale	Nutrient Benefits	Thoughts/Feelings	Behavior
		S	F	D	V	P	F				
	Total										

Exercise:

Met goal: yes/no/improving

Met all exchanges: yes/no

Exchanges to make up:

My Food Journal

Name:

Date/Day:

Daily Goal(s):

Recommended Exchanges/Consumed exchanges

Starch	Fruit	Dairy	Vegetable	Protein	Fat

Time	Food and Amount	Exchange						Hunger Scale	Nutrient Benefits	Thoughts/Feelings	Behavior
		S	F	D	V	P	F				
Total											

Exercise:

Met goal: yes/no/improving

Met all exchanges: yes/no

Exchanges to make up:

My Food Journal

Name:

Date/Day:

Daily Goal(s):

Recommended Exchanges/Consumed exchanges

Starch	Fruit	Dairy	Vegetable	Protein	Fat

Time	Food and Amount	Exchange						Hunger Scale	Nutrient Benefits	Thoughts/Feelings	Behavior
		S	F	D	V	P	F				
	Total										

Exercise:

Met goal: yes/no/improving

Met all exchanges: yes/no

Exchanges to make up:

My Food Journal

Name:

Date/Day:

Daily Goal(s):

Recommended Exchanges/Consumed exchanges

Starch	Fruit	Dairy	Vegetable	Protein	Fat

Time	Food and Amount	Exchange						Hunger Scale	Nutrient Benefits	Thoughts/Feelings	Behavior
		S	F	D	V	P	F				
	Total										

Exercise:

Met goal: yes/no/improving

Met all exchanges: yes/no

Exchanges to make up:

My Food Journal

Name:

Date/Day:

Daily Goal(s):

Recommended Exchanges/Consumed exchanges

Starch	Fruit	Dairy	Vegetable	Protein	Fat

Time	Food and Amount	Exchange					Hunger Scale	Nutrient Benefits	Thoughts/Feelings	Behavior
		S	F	D	V	P	F			
Total											

Exercise:

Met goal: yes/no/improving

Met all exchanges: yes/no

Exchanges to make up:

My Food Journal

Name: _____

Date/Day: _____ Daily Goal(s): _____

Recommended Exchanges/Consumed exchanges

Starch	Fruit	Dairy	Vegetable	Protein	Fat

Time	Food and Amount	Exchange						Hunger Scale	Nutrient Benefits	Thoughts/Feelings	Behavior
		S	F	D	V	P	F				
	Total										

Exercise: _____

Met goal: yes/no/improving

Met all exchanges: yes/no

Exchanges to make up: _____

© Copyright 2011 Amy Galena, MSH, RD, LD/N BeeNutritious

My Food Journal

Name:

Date/Day:

Daily Goal(s):

Recommended Exchanges/Consumed exchanges

Starch	Fruit	Dairy	Vegetable	Protein	Fat

Time	Food and Amount	Exchange						Hunger Scale	Nutrient Benefits	Thoughts/Feelings	Behavior
		S	F	D	V	P	F				
	Total										

Exercise:

Met goal: yes/no/improving

Met all exchanges: yes/no

Exchanges to make up:

My Food Journal

Name: _____

Date/Day: _____

Daily Goal(s): _____

Recommended Exchanges/Consumed exchanges

Starch	Fruit	Dairy	Vegetable	Protein	Fat

Time	Food and Amount	Exchange						Hunger Scale	Nutrient Benefits	Thoughts/Feelings	Behavior
		S	F	D	V	P	F				
Total											

Exercise: _____

Met goal: yes/no/improving

Met all exchanges: yes/no

Exchanges to make up: _____

My Food Journal

Name: _____

Date/Day: _____ Daily Goal(s): _____

Recommended Exchanges/Consumed exchanges

Starch	Fruit	Dairy	Vegetable	Protein	Fat

Time	Food and Amount	Exchange							Hunger Scale	Nutrient Benefits	Thoughts/Feelings	Behavior
		S	F	D	V	P	F					
Total												

Exercise: _____

Met goal: yes/no/improving

Met all exchanges: yes/no

Exchanges to make up: _____

My Food Journal

Name:

Date/Day:

Daily Goal(s):

Recommended Exchanges/Consumed exchanges

Starch	Fruit	Dairy	Vegetable	Protein	Fat

Time	Food and Amount	Exchange						Hunger Scale	Nutrient Benefits	Thoughts/Feelings	Behavior
		S	F	D	V	P	F				
Total											

Exercise:

Met goal: yes/no/improving

Met all exchanges: yes/no

Exchanges to make up:

My Food Journal

Name:

Date/Day:

Daily Goal(s):

Recommended Exchanges/Consumed exchanges

Starch	Fruit	Dairy	Vegetable	Protein	Fat

Time	Food and Amount	Exchange					Hunger Scale	Nutrient Benefits	Thoughts/Feelings	Behavior
		S	F	D	V	P	F				
Total											

Exercise:

Met goal: yes/no/improving

Met all exchanges: yes/no

Exchanges to make up:

My Food Journal

Name:

Date/Day:

Daily Goal(s):

Recommended Exchanges/Consumed exchanges

Starch		Fruit		Dairy		Vegetable		Protein		Fat	

Time	Food and Amount	Exchange						Hunger Scale	Nutrient Benefits	Thoughts/Feelings	Behavior
		S	F	D	V	P	F				
	Total										

Exercise:

Met goal: yes/no/improving

Met all exchanges: yes/no

Exchanges to make up:

My Food Journal

Name:

Date/Day:

Daily Goal(s):

Recommended Exchanges/Consumed exchanges

Starch	Fruit	Dairy	Vegetable	Protein	Fat

Time	Food and Amount	Exchange						Hunger Scale	Nutrient Benefits	Thoughts/Feelings	Behavior
		S	F	D	V	P	F				
Total											

Exercise:

Met goal: yes/no/improving

Met all exchanges: yes/no

Exchanges to make up:

My Food Journal

Name:

Date/Day: Daily Goal(s):

Recommended Exchanges/Consumed exchanges

Starch	Fruit	Dairy	Vegetable	Protein	Fat

Time	Food and Amount	Exchange						Hunger Scale	Nutrient Benefits	Thoughts/Feelings	Behavior
		S	F	D	V	P	F				
	Total										

Exercise:

Met goal: yes/no/improving

Met all exchanges: yes/no

Exchanges to make up:

My Food Journal

Name:

Date/Day:

Daily Goal(s):

Recommended Exchanges/Consumed exchanges

Starch	Fruit	Dairy	Vegetable	Protein	Fat

Time	Food and Amount	Exchange						Hunger Scale	Nutrient Benefits	Thoughts/Feelings	Behavior
		S	F	D	V	P	F				
	Total										

Exercise:

Met goal: yes/no/improving

Met all exchanges: yes/no

Exchanges to make up:

My Food Journal

Name:

Date/Day: _____ Daily Goal(s):

Recommended Exchanges/Consumed exchanges

Starch	Fruit	Dairy	Vegetable	Protein	Fat

Time	Food and Amount	Exchange						Hunger Scale	Nutrient Benefits	Thoughts/Feelings	Behavior
		S	F	D	V	P	F				
Total											

Exercise: yes/no/improving

Met goal: yes/no/improving

Met all exchanges: yes/no

Exchanges to make up:

My Food Journal

Name: _____

Date/Day: _____   Daily Goal(s): _____

Recommended Exchanges/Consumed exchanges

Starch	Fruit	Dairy	Vegetable	Protein	Fat

Time	Food and Amount	Exchange S F D V P F	Hunger Scale	Nutrient Benefits	Thoughts/Feelings	Behavior
Total						

Exercise: _____

Met goal: yes/no/improving

Met all exchanges: yes/no

Exchanges to make up: _____

My Food Journal

Name:

Date/Day:

Daily Goal(s):

Recommended Exchanges/Consumed exchanges

Starch	Fruit	Dairy	Vegetable	Protein	Fat

Time	Food and Amount	Exchange						Hunger Scale	Nutrient Benefits	Thoughts/Feelings	Behavior
		S	F	D	V	P	F				
	Total										

Exercise: yes/no/improving

Met goal: yes/no/improving

Met all exchanges: yes/no

Exchanges to make up:

My Food Journal

Name:

Date/Day:

Daily Goal(s):

Recommended Exchanges/Consumed exchanges

Starch	Fruit	Dairy	Vegetable	Protein	Fat

Time	Food and Amount	Exchange						Hunger Scale	Nutrient Benefits	Thoughts/Feelings	Behavior
		S	F	D	V	P	F				
Total											

Exercise:

Met goal: yes/no/improving

Met all exchanges: yes/no

Exchanges to make up:

My Food Journal

Name:

Date/Day:

Daily Goal(s):

Recommended Exchanges/Consumed exchanges

Starch	Fruit	Dairy	Vegetable	Protein	Fat

Time	Food and Amount	Exchange						Hunger Scale	Nutrient Benefits	Thoughts/Feelings	Behavior
		S	F	D	V	P	F				
Total											

Exercise:

Met goal: yes/no/improving

Met all exchanges: yes/no

Exchanges to make up:

My Food Journal

Name: _____

Date/Day: _____   Daily Goal(s): _____

Recommended Exchanges/Consumed exchanges

Starch	Fruit	Dairy	Vegetable	Protein	Fat

Time	Food and Amount	Exchange						Hunger Scale	Nutrient Benefits	Thoughts/Feelings	Behavior
		S	F	D	V	P	F				
Total											

Exercise: _____

Met goal: yes/no/improving

Met all exchanges: yes/no

Exchanges to make up: _____

My Food Journal

Name:

Date/Day: Daily Goal(s):

Recommended Exchanges/Consumed exchanges

Starch	Fruit	Dairy	Vegetable	Protein	Fat

Time	Food and Amount	Exchange						Hunger Scale	Nutrient Benefits	Thoughts/Feelings	Behavior
		S	F	D	V	P	F				
Total											

Exercise:

Met goal: yes/no/improving

Met all exchanges: yes/no

Exchanges to make up:

My Food Journal

Name: _____

Date/Day: _____   Daily Goal(s): _____

Recommended Exchanges/Consumed exchanges

Starch	Fruit	Dairy	Vegetable	Protein	Fat

Time	Food and Amount	Exchange						Hunger Scale	Nutrient Benefits	Thoughts/Feelings	Behavior
		S	F	D	V	P	F				
	Total										

Exercise: _____

Met goal: yes/no/improving

Met all exchanges: yes/no

Exchanges to make up:

My Food Journal

Name:

Date/Day:

Daily Goal(s):

Recommended Exchanges/Consumed exchanges

Starch	Fruit	Dairy	Vegetable	Protein	Fat

Time	Food and Amount	Exchange						Hunger Scale	Nutrient Benefits	Thoughts/Feelings	Behavior
		S	F	D	V	P	F				
Total											

Exercise:

Met goal: yes/no/improving

Met all exchanges: yes/no

Exchanges to make up:

My Food Journal

Name: _____

Date/Day: _____ Daily Goal(s): _____

Recommended Exchanges/Consumed exchanges

	Starch	Fruit	Dairy	Vegetable	Protein	Fat

Time	Food and Amount	Exchange						Hunger Scale	Nutrient Benefits	Thoughts/Feelings	Behavior
		S	F	D	V	P	F				
	Total										

Exercise: _____

Met goal: yes/no/improving

Met all exchanges: yes/no

Exchanges to make up: _____

My Food Journal

Name:

Date/Day:

Recommended Exchanges/Consumed exchanges

Starch	Fruit	Dairy	Vegetable	Protein	Fat

Daily Goal(s):

Time	Food and Amount	Exchange						Hunger Scale	Nutrient Benefits	Thoughts/Feelings	Behavior
		S	F	D	V	P	F				
	Total										

Exercise:

Met goal: yes/no/improving

Met all exchanges: yes/no

Exchanges to make up:

My Food Journal

Name:

Date/Day: _____ **Daily Goal(s):**

Recommended Exchanges/Consumed exchanges

Starch	Fruit	Dairy	Vegetable	Protein	Fat

Time	Food and Amount	Exchange						Hunger Scale	Nutrient Benefits	Thoughts/Feelings	Behavior
		S	F	D	V	P	F				
	Total										

Exercise:

Met goal: yes/no/improving

Met all exchanges: yes/no

Exchanges to make up:

My Food Journal

Name:

Date/Day: Daily Goal(s):

Recommended Exchanges/Consumed exchanges

Starch	Fruit	Dairy	Vegetable	Protein	Fat

Time	Food and Amount	Exchange							Hunger Scale	Nutrient Benefits	Thoughts/Feelings	Behavior
		S	F	D	V	P	F					
	Total											

Exercise:

Met goal: yes/no/improving

Met all exchanges: yes/no

Exchanges to make up:

My Food Journal

Name:

Date/Day:

Daily Goal(s):

Recommended Exchanges/Consumed exchanges

Starch	Fruit	Dairy	Vegetable	Protein	Fat

Time	Food and Amount	Exchange							Hunger Scale	Nutrient Benefits	Thoughts/Feelings	Behavior
		S	F	D	V	P	F					
Total												

Exercise:

Met goal: yes/no/improving

Met all exchanges: yes/no

Exchanges to make up:

My Food Journal

Name:

Date/Day:

Daily Goal(s):

Recommended Exchanges/Consumed exchanges

Starch	Fruit	Dairy	Vegetable	Protein	Fat

Time	Food and Amount	Exchange						Hunger Scale	Nutrient Benefits	Thoughts/Feelings	Behavior
		S	F	D	V	P	F				
	Total										

Exercise:

Met goal: yes/no/improving

Met all exchanges: yes/no

Exchanges to make up:

My Food Journal

Name:

Date/Day:

Daily Goal(s):

Recommended Exchanges/Consumed exchanges

Starch	Fruit	Dairy	Vegetable	Protein	Fat

Time	Food and Amount	Exchange					Hunger Scale	Nutrient Benefits	Thoughts/Feelings	Behavior
		S	F	D	V	P	F				
	Total										

Exercise:

Met goal: yes/no/improving

Met all exchanges: yes/no

Exchanges to make up:

My Food Journal

Name: _____

Date/Day: _____ Daily Goal(s): _____

Recommended Exchanges/Consumed exchanges

Starch	Fruit	Dairy	Vegetable	Protein	Fat

Time	Food and Amount	Exchange						Hunger Scale	Nutrient Benefits	Thoughts/Feelings	Behavior
		S	F	D	V	P	F				
	Total										

Exercise: _____

Met goal: yes/no/improving

Met all exchanges: yes/no

Exchanges to make up: _____

My Food Journal

Name:

Date/Day:

Daily Goal(s):

Recommended Exchanges/Consumed exchanges

Starch	Fruit	Dairy	Vegetable	Protein	Fat

Time	Food and Amount	Exchange						Hunger Scale	Nutrient Benefits	Thoughts/Feelings	Behavior
		S	F	D	V	P	F				
	Total										

Exercise:

Met goal: yes/no/improving

Met all exchanges: yes/no

Exchanges to make up:

My Food Journal

Name:

Date/Day:

Daily Goal(s):

Recommended Exchanges/Consumed exchanges

Starch	Fruit	Dairy	Vegetable	Protein	Fat

Time	Food and Amount	Exchange							Hunger Scale	Nutrient Benefits	Thoughts/Feelings	Behavior
		S	F	D	V	U	F					
	Total											

Exercise:

Met goal: yes/no/improving

Met all exchanges: yes/no

Exchanges to make up:

My Food Journal

Name:

Date/Day:

Daily Goal(s):

Recommended Exchanges/Consumed exchanges

Starch	Fruit	Dairy	Vegetable	Protein	Fat

Time	Food and Amount	Exchange						Hunger Scale	Nutrient Benefits	Thoughts/Feelings	Behavior
		S	F	D	V	P	F				
Total											

Exercise:

Met goal: yes/no/improving

Met all exchanges: yes/no

Exchanges to make up:

My Food Journal

Name:

Date/Day:

Daily Goal(s):

Recommended Exchanges/Consumed exchanges

Starch	Fruit	Dairy	Vegetable	Protein	Fat

Time	Food and Amount	Exchange							Hunger Scale	Nutrient Benefits	Thoughts/Feelings	Behavior
		S	F	D	V	P	F					
	Total											

Exercise:

Met goal: yes/no/improving

Met all exchanges: yes/no

Exchanges to make up:

My Food Journal

Name:

Date/Day:

Daily Goal(s):

Recommended Exchanges/Consumed exchanges

Starch	Fruit	Dairy	Vegetable	Protein	Fat

Time	Food and Amount	Exchange						Hunger Scale	Nutrient Benefits	Thoughts/Feelings	Behavior
		S	F	D	V	P	F				
	Total										

Exercise:

Met goal: yes/no/improving

Met all exchanges: yes/no

Exchanges to make up:

My Food Journal

Name:

Date/Day: Daily Goal(s):

Recommended Exchanges/Consumed exchanges

Starch	Fruit	Dairy	Vegetable	Protein	Fat

Time	Food and Amount	Exchange							Hunger Scale	Nutrient Benefits	Thoughts/Feelings	Behavior
		S	F	D	V	P	F					
Total												

Exercise:

Met goal: yes/no/improving

Met all exchanges: yes/no

Exchanges to make up:

My Food Journal

Name:

Date/Day:

Daily Goal(s):

Recommended Exchanges/Consumed exchanges

Starch	Fruit	Dairy	Vegetable	Protein	Fat

Time	Food and Amount	Exchange							Hunger Scale	Nutrient Benefits	Thoughts/Feelings	Behavior
		S	F	D	V	P	F					
Total												

Exercise:

Met goal: yes/no/improving

Met all exchanges: yes/no

Exchanges to make up:

My Food Journal

Name:

Date/Day: Daily Goal(s):

Recommended Exchanges/Consumed exchanges

Starch	Fruit	Dairy	Vegetable	Protein	Fat

Time	Food and Amount	Exchange						Hunger Scale	Nutrient Benefits	Thoughts/Feelings	Behavior
		S	F	D	V	P	F				
	Total										

Exercise:

Met goal: yes/no/improving

Met all exchanges: yes/no

Exchanges to make up:

© Copyright 2011 Amy Galena, MSH, RD, LD/N BeeNutritious

My Food Journal

Name:

Date/Day:

Daily Goal(s):

Recommended Exchanges/Consumed exchanges

Starch	Fruit	Dairy	Vegetable	Protein	Fat

Time	Food and Amount	Exchange						Hunger Scale	Nutrient Benefits	Thoughts/Feelings	Behavior
		S	F	D	V	P	F				
	Total										

Met all exchanges: yes/no

Exchanges to make up:

Exercise:

Met goal: yes/no/improving

My Food Journal

Name:

Date/Day:

Daily Goal(s):

Recommended Exchanges/Consumed exchanges

Starch	Fruit	Dairy	Vegetable	Protein	Fat

Time	Food and Amount	Exchange					Hunger Scale	Nutrient Benefits	Thoughts/Feelings	Behavior
		S	F	D	V	P	F				
	Total										

Exercise:

Met goal: yes/no/improving

Met all exchanges: yes/no

Exchanges to make up:

My Food Journal

Name: _____

Date/Day: _____

Daily Goal(s): _____

Recommended Exchanges/Consumed exchanges

Starch	Fruit	Dairy	Vegetable	Protein	Fat

Time	Food and Amount	Exchange							Hunger Scale	Nutrient Benefits	Thoughts/Feelings	Behavior
		S	F	D	V	P	F					
Total												

Exercise: _____

Met goal: yes/no/improving

Met all exchanges: yes/no

Exchanges to make up: _____

My Food Journal

Name:

Date/Day:

Daily Goal(s):

Recommended Exchanges/Consumed exchanges

Starch	Fruit	Dairy	Vegetable	Protein	Fat

Time	Food and Amount	Exchange							Hunger Scale	Nutrient Benefits	Thoughts/Feelings	Behavior
		S	F	D	V	P	F					
Total												

Exercise:

Met goal: yes/no/improving

Met all exchanges: yes/no

Exchanges to make up:

© Copyright 2011 Amy Galena, MSH, RD, LD/N BeeNutritious

My Food Journal

Name:

Date/Day: Daily Goal(s):

Recommended Exchanges/Consumed exchanges

Starch	Fruit	Dairy	Vegetable	Protein	Fat

Time	Food and Amount	Exchange						Hunger Scale	Nutrient Benefits	Thoughts/Feelings	Behavior
		S	F	D	V	P	F				
	Total										

Exercise:

Met goal: yes/no/improving

Met all exchanges: yes/no

Exchanges to make up:

My Food Journal

Name:

Date/Day:

Daily Goal(s):

Recommended Exchanges/Consumed exchanges

Starch	Fruit	Dairy	Vegetable	Protein	Fat

Time	Food and Amount	Exchange						Hunger Scale	Nutrient Benefits	Thoughts/Feelings	Behavior
		S	F	D	V	P	F				
	Total										

Exercise:

Met goal: yes/no/improving

Met all exchanges: yes/no

Exchanges to make up:

© Copyright 2011 Amy Galena, MSH, RD, LD/N BeeNutritious

My Food Journal

Name:

Date/Day:

Daily Goal(s):

Recommended Exchanges/Consumed exchanges

Starch	Fruit	Dairy	Vegetable	Protein	Fat

Time	Food and Amount	Exchange						Hunger Scale	Nutrient Benefits	Thoughts/Feelings	Behavior
		S	F	D	V	P	F				
Total											

Exercise:

Met goal: yes/no/improving

Met all exchanges: yes/no

Exchanges to make up:

My Food Journal

Name:

Date/Day: Daily Goal(s):

Recommended Exchanges/Consumed exchanges

Starch	Fruit	Dairy	Vegetable	Protein	Fat

Time	Food and Amount	Exchange						Hunger Scale	Nutrient Benefits	Thoughts/Feelings	Behavior
		S	F	D	V	P	F				
	Total										

Exercise:

Met goal: yes/no/improving

Met all exchanges: yes/no

Exchanges to make up:

My Food Journal

Name:

Date/Day:

Daily Goal(s):

Recommended Exchanges/Consumed exchanges

Starch	Fruit	Dairy	Vegetable	Protein	Fat

Time	Food and Amount	Exchange						Hunger Scale	Nutrient Benefits	Thoughts/Feelings	Behavior
		S	F	D	V	P	F				
	Total										

Exercise:

Met goal: yes/no/improving

Met all exchanges: yes/no

Exchanges to make up:

My Food Journal

Name:

Date/Day:

Daily Goal(s):

Recommended Exchanges/Consumed exchanges

Starch	Fruit	Dairy	Vegetable	Protein	Fat

Time	Food and Amount	Exchange						Hunger Scale	Nutrient Benefits	Thoughts/Feelings	Behavior
		S	F	D	V	P	F				
Total											

Exercise:

Met goal: yes/no/improving

Met all exchanges: yes/no

Exchanges to make up:

My Food Journal

Name:

Date/Day: _____ **Daily Goal(s):**

Recommended Exchanges/Consumed exchanges

Starch	Fruit	Dairy	Vegetable	Protein	Fat

Time	Food and Amount	Exchange						Hunger Scale	Nutrient Benefits	Thoughts/Feelings	Behavior
		S	F	D	V	P	F				
Total											

Exercise:

Met goal: yes/no/improving

Met all exchanges: yes/no

Exchanges to make up:

My Food Journal

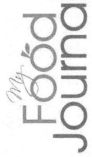

Name:

Date/Day:

Daily Goal(s):

Recommended Exchanges/Consumed exchanges

Starch	Fruit	Dairy	Vegetable	Protein	Fat

Time	Food and Amount	Exchange						Hunger Scale	Nutrient Benefits	Thoughts/Feelings	Behavior
		S	F	D	V	P	F				
	Total										

Exercise:

Met goal: yes/no/improving

Met all exchanges: yes/no

Exchanges to make up:

My Food Journal

Name:

Date/Day: Daily Goal(s):

Recommended Exchanges/Consumed exchanges

Starch	Fruit	Dairy	Vegetable	Protein	Fat

Time	Food and Amount	Exchange						Hunger Scale	Nutrient Benefits	Thoughts/Feelings	Behavior
		S	F	D	V	P	F				
Total											

Exercise:

Met goal: yes/no/improving

Met all exchanges: yes/no

Exchanges to make up:

My Food Journal

Name:

Date/Day:

Daily Goal(s):

Recommended Exchanges/Consumed exchanges

Starch	Fruit	Dairy	Vegetable	Protein	Fat

Time	Food and Amount	Exchange							Hunger Scale	Nutrient Benefits	Thoughts/Feelings	Behavior
		S	F	D	V	P	F					
	Total											

Exercise:

Met goal: yes/no/improving

Met all exchanges: yes/no

Exchanges to make up:

My Food Journal

Name:

Date/Day:

Daily Goal(s):

Recommended Exchanges/Consumed exchanges

Starch	Fruit	Dairy	Vegetable	Protein	Fat

Time	Food and Amount	Exchange					Hunger Scale	Nutrient Benefits	Thoughts/Feelings	Behavior
		S	F	D	V	P	F				
Total											

Exercise:

Met goal: yes/no/improving

Met all exchanges: yes/no

Exchanges to make up:

© Copyright 2011 Amy Galena, MSH, RD, LD/N BeeNutritious

My Food Journal

Name:

Date/Day:

Daily Goal(s):

Recommended Exchanges/Consumed exchanges

Starch	Fruit	Dairy	Vegetable	Protein	Fat

Time	Food and Amount	Exchange						Hunger Scale	Nutrient Benefits	Thoughts/Feelings	Behavior
		S	F	D	V	P	F				
	Total										

Exercise:

Met goal: yes/no/improving

Met all exchanges: yes/no

Exchanges to make up:

© Copyright 2011 Amy Galena, MSH, RD, LD/N BeeNutritious

My Food Journal

Name:

Date/Day:

Daily Goal(s):

Recommended Exchanges/Consumed exchanges

Starch	Fruit	Dairy	Vegetable	Protein	Fat

Time	Food and Amount	Exchange					Hunger Scale	Nutrient Benefits	Thoughts/Feelings	Behavior
		S	F	D	V	P	F				
Total											

Exercise:

Met goal: yes/no/improving

Met all exchanges: yes/no

Exchanges to make up:

My Food Journal

Name: _____

Date/Day: _____   Daily Goal(s): _____

Recommended Exchanges/Consumed exchanges

Starch	Fruit	Dairy	Vegetable	Protein	Fat

Time	Food and Amount	Exchange						Hunger Scale	Nutrient Benefits	Thoughts/Feelings	Behavior
		S	F	D	V	P	F				
	Total										

Exercise: _____

Met goal: yes/no/improving

Met all exchanges: yes/no

Exchanges to make up: _____

My Food Journal

Name:

Date/Day:

Daily Goal(s):

Recommended Exchanges/Consumed exchanges

Starch	Fruit	Dairy	Vegetable	Protein	Fat

Time	Food and Amount	Exchange						Hunger Scale	Nutrient Benefits	Thoughts/Feelings	Behavior
		S	F	D	V	P	F				
	Total										

Exercise:

Met goal: yes/no/improving

Met all exchanges: yes/no

Exchanges to make up:

My Food Journal

Name:

Date/Day:

Daily Goal(s):

Recommended Exchanges/Consumed exchanges

Starch	Fruit	Dairy	Vegetable	Protein	Fat

Time	Food and Amount	Exchange						Hunger Scale	Nutrient Benefits	Thoughts/Feelings	Behavior
		S	F	D	V	P	F				
Total											

Exercise: yes/no/improving

Met goal: yes/no/improving

Met all exchanges: yes/no

Exchanges to make up:

© Copyright 2011 Amy Galena, MSH, RD, LD/N BeeNutritious

My Food Journal

Name:

Date/Day:

Daily Goal(s):

Recommended Exchanges/Consumed exchanges

Starch	Fruit	Dairy	Vegetable	Protein	Fat

Time	Food and Amount	Exchange						Hunger Scale	Nutrient Benefits	Thoughts/Feelings	Behavior
		S	F	D	V	P	F				
Total											

Exercise:

Met goal: yes/no/improving

Met all exchanges: yes/no

Exchanges to make up:

JOURNAL PAGES

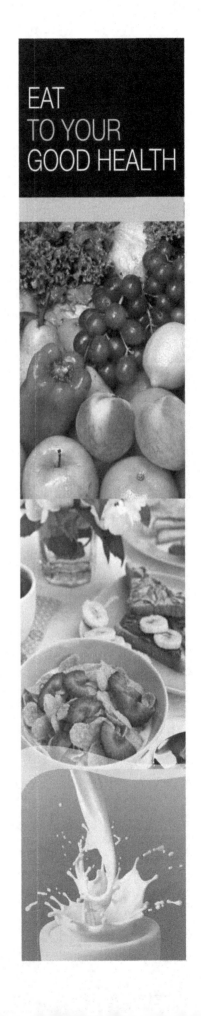

EAT
TO YOUR
GOOD HEALTH

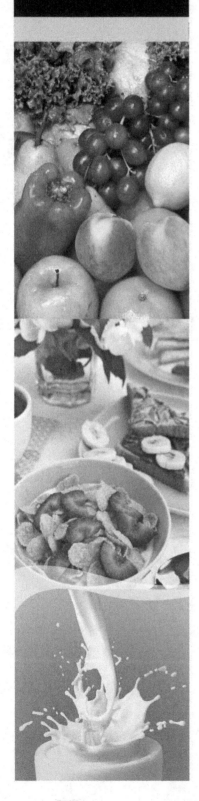

EAT
TO YOUR
GOOD HEALTH

INDEX

INDEX

V

W

Y

Z